W9-AYA-587

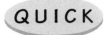

Reference to
CRITICAL CARE

• •

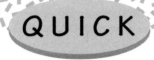

QUICK

Reference to
CRITICAL CARE

• •

NANCY H. DIEPENBROCK, RN, CCRN

Staff Nurse
Intensive Care Unit
Zale Lipshy University Hospital
Dallas, Texas

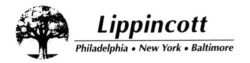

Lippincott
Philadelphia • New York • Baltimore

Acquisitions Editor: Susan M. Glover, RN, MSN
Assistant Editor: Bridget Blatteau
Project Editor: Gretchen Metzger
Senior Production Manager: Helen Ewan
Production Coordinator: Michael Carcel
Assistant Art Director: Kathy Kelley-Luedtke

9 8 7 6 5 4 3

                     Library of Congress Cataloging-in-Publications Data
Diepenbrock, Nancy H.
    Quick reference to critical care / Nancy H. Diepenbrock.
    p. cm.
    Includes index.
    ISBN 0-7817-1862-7 (alk. paper)
    1. Critical care medicine—Handbooks, manuals, etc. I. Title.
RC86.8 .D54 1999
                                          98-44543
                                          CIP

Care has been taken to confirm the accuracy of the information presented and to describe generally accepted practices. However, the authors,
editors, and publisher are not responsible for errors or omissions or for
any consequences from application of the information in this book and
make no warranty, express or implied, with respect to the contents of
the publication.

The authors, editors, and publisher have exerted every effort to ensure
that drug selection and dosage set forth in this text are in accordance
with current recommendations and practice at the time of publication.
However, in view of ongoing research, changes in government regula-
tions, and the constant flow of information relating to drug therapy and
drug reactions, the reader is urged to check the package insert for each
drug for any change in indications and dosage and for added warnings
and precautions. This is particularly important when the recommended
agent is a new or infrequently employed drug.

Some drugs and medical devices presented in this publication have
Food and Drug Administration (FDA) clearance for limited use in re-
stricted research settings. It is the responsibility of the health care provider
to ascertain the FDA status of each drug or device planned for use in
their clinical practice.

*To my peers, who made me do it;
and for David,
who made it possible.*

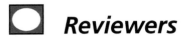

Reviewers

Janet L. Gysi, RN, MA, CCRN

Instructor
Nursing
Iowa Wesleyan College
Mount Pleasant, Iowa

Staff Nurse
Emergency Treatment Center
Burlington Medical Center
Burlington, Iowa

Darlene A. Petersen, RN, MSN, CNS, CCRN

Critical Care Clinical Nurse Specialist
Cardiology Division
Memorial Hospital at Gulfport
Gulfport, Mississippi

Linda Valenti, RN, CCRN

Staff Nurse
Cooper Hospital
Camden, New Jersey

Preface

Anyone involved in the care of the critically ill has, no doubt, at some time experienced the frustration of a memory lapse when it came to a minute detail of clinical practice. Such occurrences led to the evolution of this book, with the momentum to have it published coming from nurses, residents, and students alike all voicing the common and serious concern that they "can't remember everything!"

This book deals with quick facts and quick solutions. Its purpose is to serve as a memory jogger when time is crucial, leaving detailed clinical information to an in-depth textbook. It is organized into an easy-to-use format, with the addition of a host of anagrams, hints, tables, and charts to assist the user to recall otherwise difficult-to-remember material. The content is divided into chapters by organ system and reference base, and for ease of use and quick access, topics are organized alphabetically within each chapter. Extensive cross-referencing is included, to avoid any discrepancy among terms, and an in-depth index is included to guide the user to the proper chapter. The text features extra space to encourage the user to add notes of personal interest or those specific to institution practices, and headings in bold make it easier to scan the pages for specific data. Chapters 1 through 7 relate specifically to body systems: 1-Neurologic; 2-Cardiovascular; 3-Pulmonary; 4-Gastrointestinal/Urinary; 5-Renal; 6-Endocrine; 7-Hematologic/Immune. Chapters 8 through 11 focus on specific critical care facts: 8-Drugs, Doses, Tables; 9-Conversions, Calculations, Compatability; 10-Labs; 11-Miscellaneous.

ACKNOWLEDGMENTS

The author gratefully acknowledges those individuals who took time from their own busy schedules to review the text and make suggestions: Dr. Cole A. Giller, for his insights in the neurologic chapter; Dr. Rick A. Lange, for his guidance with the cardiovascular chapter; Dr. John E. Fitzgerald, for his invaluable help with the pulmonary chapter; and Jeff Frye, PharmD, for his assistance and diligent research on the drugs and conversions chapters. Thanks also to Kim McCasland for her help in the typing of the manuscript, her knowledge in the use of the computer, and her unending encouragement.

Nancy H. Diepenbrock, RN, CCRN

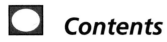

Contents

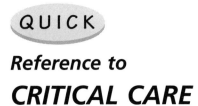

QUICK

Reference to
CRITICAL CARE

· ·

Neurologic System

◖ ACCOMMODATION

Accommodation is the adaptation of eyes for near vision. It is demonstrated by having patient focus on object at arm's length. When object is brought toward patient, the pupils should converge and constrict. This cannot be done on a comatose patient.

◖ ACOUSTIC NEUROMA (see Tumors, Neurogenic)

◖ ADENOMA (see Tumors, Neurogenic)

◖ AMYOTROPHIC LATERAL SCLEROSIS (see also Spinal Cord)

Progressive wasting, weakness, and spasticity of muscles of amyotrophic lateral sclerosis is due to a combination of upper and lower motor neuron damage. Wasting and weakness are related to *lower* motor neuron damage; spasticity and exaggerated weakness are related to *upper* motor neuron damage.

⬤ ANATOMY: ARTERIAL BLOOD SUPPLY TO BRAIN

Area supplied by
anterior cerebral artery

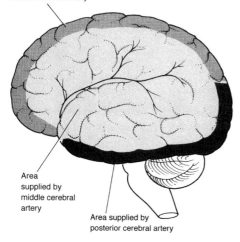

Area
supplied by
middle cerebral
artery

Area supplied by
posterior cerebral artery

FIGURE 1-1 Arterial blood supply to the brain.

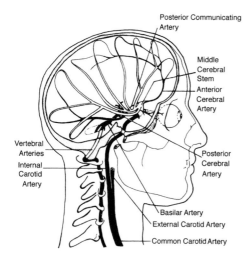

Posterior Communicating
Artery

Middle
Cerebral
Stem

Anterior
Cerebral
Artery

Vertebral
Arteries

Internal
Carotid
Artery

Posterior
Cerebral
Artery

Basilar Artery

External Carotid Artery

Common Carotid Artery

FIGURE 1-2 Major blood vessels to the brain. The internal, carotid, anterior, and middle cerebral arteries constitute the anterior circulation. The vertebral, basilar, and posterior cerebral arteries and branches make up the posterior circulation.

○ ANATOMY: CRANIAL LAYERS

Remember the mnemonic: ⒺⒹ'Ⓢ Ⓐ ⓈuperⓅizza Ⓜan

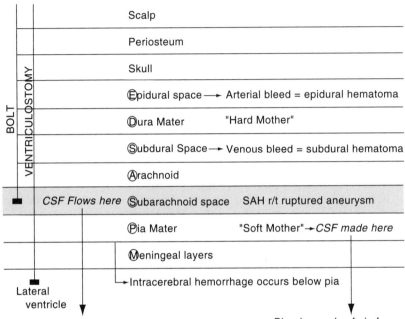

Scalp	
Periosteum	
Skull	
Ⓔpidural space ⟶	Arterial bleed = epidural hematoma
Ⓓura Mater	"Hard Mother"
Ⓢubdural Space ⟶	Venous bleed = subdural hematoma
Ⓐrachnoid	
CSF Flows here Ⓢubarachnoid space	SAH r/t ruptured aneurysm
Ⓟia Mater	"Soft Mother" ⟶ *CSF made here*
Ⓜeningeal layers	

BOLT

VENTRICULOSTOMY

CSF Flows here

└⟶ Intracerebral hemorrhage occurs below pia

■ Lateral ventricle

CSF circulates from ventricles in brain, around SA space, around brain, around spinal cord, through villi into dural sinuses for absorption

Blood vessels of pia form choroid plexus, a special capillary bed that filters blood so as blood passes through it, it becomes CSF (See Cerebrospinal Fluid)

FIGURE 1-3 Cranial layers.

N O T E S

⬤ **ANEURYSMS (see also Subarachnoid Hemorrhage, Vasospasm)**

Numerous subarachnoid grading scales have been proposed; however, the Hunt and Hess scale is the most widely used:

To OR for clip. Good prognosis.
- Grade 0 = Unruptured aneurysm.
- Grade 1 = Minimal bleed. Slight headache, slight nuchal rigidity. No neurologic deficits.
- Grade 2 = Mild bleed. Awake, alert with mild headache. Neck rigid. Possible third nerve palsy.
- Grade 3 = Moderate bleed. Drowsy. Neck rigid. Mild focal deficits.

Wait until grade improves. Treat ↑ ICP. Poor prognosis.
- Grade 4 = Moderate to severe bleed. Unresponsive. Mild to severe hemiparesis. Neck rigid. Possible early decerebration.
- Grade 5 = Severe bleed. Deep coma. Decerebrate rigidity.

- **Rebleed risk:** Peak incidence occurs 24 to 48 hours following initial bleed. Approximately 30% to 40% of patients rebleed within first several weeks, with mortality rate of 42%.
- **Survival:** On average, 25% die the first day, and 50% die within the first 3 months; 50% of survivors have major deficits.
- **Sites:** About 85% of aneurysms are located anteriorly. This is good because the posterior area is difficult to access.
- **Size:**
  - Super giant >50 mm
  - Giant 25 to 50 mm
  - Large 15 to 25 mm
  - Small <15 mm
- **Types:**
  - Berry: Most common. Rounded with a neck or stem; looks like "berries."
  - Saccular: Any aneurysm having a saccular outpouching.
  - Fusiform: Diffuse enlargement of arterial wall. No neck or stem; looks like a balloon. Usually does not cause SAH.
  - Charcot-Bouchard: Origin is basal ganglia or brain stem. Microscopic formations related to hypertension.
  - Mycotic: Rare; caused by septic emboli which separate endothelial lining; related to bacterial endocarditis.

(continued)

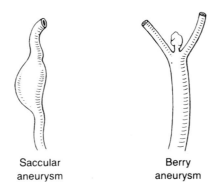

Saccular
aneurysm

Berry
aneurysm

FIGURE 1-4 Saccular and berry aneurysms.

■ **Surgical intervention:** Clipping or ligation of the aneurysm neck provides the best protection against rebleeding, although the initial risk may be slightly higher.

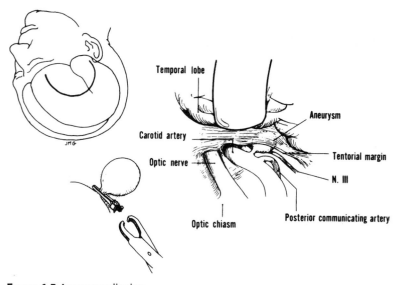

Temporal lobe

Aneurysm

Carotid artery

Tentorial margin

Optic nerve

N. III

Posterior communicating artery

Optic chiasm

FIGURE 1-5 Aneurysm clipping.

⬤ **APNEUSTIC BREATHING (see Respiratory Patterns in Part 3, Pulmonary System)**

⬤ **ARTERIOVENOUS MALFORMATION**

Arteriovenous malformations (AVMs) are congenital brain lesions composed of tangled, dilated vessels that form an abnormal communication

(*continued*)

between arterial and venous systems. Intracranial "steal" occurs when the AVM is large, related to blood being diverted from one area of brain tissue because of lower vascularization in another area.

- **Signs and symptoms:** Seizure activity is most common. Hemorrhage and/or headache occur in about 50% of patients.
- **Treatment:** Similar to aneurysms, though AVMs pose less risk of bleed with intervention.
  1. Embolization
  2. Surgical excision
  3. Gamma knife, linear accelerator, or proton beam radiation (for surgically inaccessible AVMs)

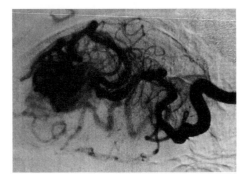

FIGURE 1-6 Arteriovenous malformation.

◯ BABINSKI'S REFLEX

Positive response for Babinski's reflex is fanning of toes and extension of great toes with stimulation of plantar surface of foot. It is normal in babies, but abnormal in adults. Response is related to upper motor neuron lesion and is seen on opposite side of cerebral damage.

Negative response is flexion of foot and is normal in adults.

◯ BASILAR SKULL FRACTURE

Injury to olfactory (first cranial) nerve is common with fracture, along with otorrhea or rhinorrhea. Drainage sample may be positive for glucose, though this is not always a reliable sign. Allow CSF to drain freely. Avoid NG, nasal suction, Valsalva's maneuver, cough. Raccoon eyes, which are ecchymotic areas around the eye orbits, indicate an anterior fossa fracture. Battle's sign, which is ecchymosis over the mastoid bone, is also present.

◯ BATTLE'S SIGN (see Basilar Skull Fracture)

⬤ **BIOT'S RESPIRATIONS (see Respiratory Patterns in Part 3, Pulmonary System)**

⬤ **BLOOD-BRAIN BARRIER (see also Choroid Plexus, Anatomy: Cranial Layers)**

Blood-brain barrier refers to the special permeability of brain capillaries and choroid plexus that limits transfer of certain substances into extracellular fluid of CSF of brain. H_2O, CO_2, O_2, and glucose cross easily. It is important because the blood-brain barrier is often damaged or infected when tissue is injured; damage leads to increased permeability.

⬤ **BRAIN DEATH CRITERIA***

Brain death diagnosis is made in the absence of hypothermia (temperature $<32.2°C$) and central nervous system depressants. Patient must be:

1. Areflexic except for simple spinal cord reflexes; pupillary, extraocular, corneal, gag, and cough reflexes are absent.

2. Without spontaneous respiration as determined by apnea test.
    To do an apnea test: Preoxygenate patient. Disconnect ventilator, and give O_2 at 8–12 L/min by tracheal cannula. Observe patient for spontaneous respirations. After 10 minutes, draw ABGs. PCO_2 must be >60 mmHg for an accurate test. Reconnect the ventilator. Patient is considered apneic if PCO_2 is >60 mmHg and there is no respiratory movement. If hypotension and/or arrhythmia develop, reconnect ventilator. Consider other confirmatory tests.

3. Considered to have an irreversible condition. Duration of observation depends on clinical judgment: 12 hours is recommended when an irreversible condition is well established and no confirmatory test; 24 hours is recommended for anoxic brain damage and no confirmatory test.

4. Positive for flat EEG (if performed).

5. Positive for absence of blood flow by cerebral radionuclide scan or arteriogram (if performed).

⬤ **BRAIN STEM (see also Cranial Nerve Exam)**

Brain stem collectively includes midbrain, pons, medulla. It is an area that controls basic functions dealing largely with involuntary activities, *(continued)*

Criteria are from the President's Commission for the Study of Ethical Problems in Medicine and Biomedical and Behavioral Research.

that is, blood pressure, heart rate, respirations. Brain stem is "bottommost" in skull. Brain stem "trouble" can be identified by means of cranial nerve tests (see Cranial Nerve Exam).

◐ BRAIN TUMORS (see Tumors, Neurogenic)

◐ BREATHING PATTERNS (see Respiratory Patterns in Part 3, Pulmonary System)

◐ BROWN-SÉQUARD'S SYNDROME

Syndrome is due to incomplete lesion to one side of spinal cord, related to trauma.

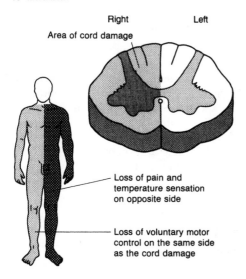

Right   Left

Area of cord damage

Loss of pain and temperature sensation on opposite side

Loss of voluntary motor control on the same side as the cord damage

FIGURE 1-7 Brown-Séquard's syndrome.

REMEMBER: Whatever side the lesion is on (right or left), the lesion causes **that side** to **lose motor function.** The opposite side loses pain and temperature sensation.

◐ BRUDZINSKI'S SIGN (see also Kernig's Sign)

Hip, knees flex in response to passive flexion of neck, known as Brudzinski's sign. Sign is positive in meningitis, positive in bleeding into subarachnoid space.

◯ CALORIC TEST (see also Doll's Eyes)

This tests the oculovestibular reflex, eighth cranial nerve. It helps evaluate the integrity of the brain stem. It is used only with patients in deep coma and with absent doll's eyes (see also Doll's Eyes). Patient is supine with head of bed up 30°. About 5 to 10 mL of ice water is instilled tympanically. Normal response (meaning pathways intact) is evidenced by conjugate deviation of both eyes to the direction of the ice water stimulus. Brain stem says, "Hey, what's that cold?" and looks toward it. The eye deviation is then followed by rapid nystagmus. An abnormal response is indicated by a dysconjugate gaze, or no eye movement at all.

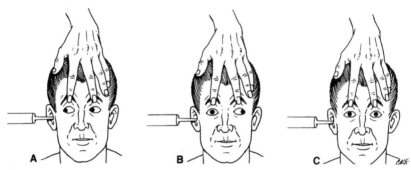

FIGURE 1-8 Caloric test. **(A)** Normal response—ice water in the ear produces conjugate eye movements followed by rapid nystagmus. **(B)** and **(C)** Abnormal response—infusion produces dysconjugate or asymmetrical eye movements or no eye movements at all.

◯ CENTRAL HERNIATION (see Herniation)

◯ CENTRAL NEUROGENIC HYPERVENTILATION (see Respiratory Patterns in Part 3, Pulmonary System)

◯ CEREBRAL PALSY

Cerebral palsy is a disease of the upper motor neurons causing spasticity.

NOTES

⬤ **CEREBRAL PERFUSION PRESSURE** (see also Increased Intracranial Pressure, Intracranial Pressure Monitoring)

Cerebral perfusion pressure (CPP) refers to the pressure difference across the brain between incoming mean arterial pressure and the opposing intracranial pressure:

CPP	MAP minus ICP
Average CPP	80 to 100 mmHg
Minimum for perfusion	50 mmHg
Brain death	<30 mmHg

⬤ **CEREBROSPINAL FLUID** (see also Anatomy: Cranial Layers, Halo Sign, Lumbar Puncture, Spinal Cord)

Cerebrospinal fluid (CSF) is made in lateral ventricles by choroid plexus. It is constantly produced and constantly absorbed. It circulates from ventricles in brain, around subarachnoid space and spinal cord. It is absorbed through villi into dura mater. Approximately 400 to 500 cc of CSF is made daily, or about 20 cc/hr. About 15 to 25 cc is located in each ventricle. It is characteristically clear and colorless (xanthrochromic CSF is sign of bleeding in area), with pressure of 80 to 180 mm H_2O while patient is side lying.

Abnormal lab values for CSF:

The following are "rules of thumb" only.

- **RBCs:** Finding RBCs in the CSF indicates hemorrhage somewhere in the central nervous system, for example, from torn or ruptured blood vessels from injury or ruptured aneurysm. This can also be due to a bloody spinal tap.

- **Increased cells:** Increased cells may indicate infection somewhere in the central nervous system. For example, polymorphonuclear leukocytes and increased lymphocytes may occur with viral infections and tuberculosis. If extremely large numbers of cells are present, the CSF may appear cloudy.

- **Lowered blood sugar:** This often results from bacterial infections of the central nervous system or due to a subarachnoid hemorrhage. A normal glucose value for CSF is 60% of serum glucose.

- **Lowered chloride level:** Drop in chloride often results from bacterial infections of the central nervous system.

- **Increased protein level:** Rise in protein usually occurs in the presence of a brain tumor or degenerative disease.

(continued)

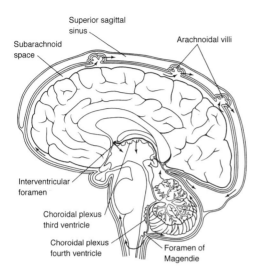

FIGURE 1-9 Flow of cerebrospinal fluid from the time of its formation from blood in the choroid plexuses, until its return to the blood in the superior sagittal sinus.

⬤ **CHEYNE-STOKES RESPIRATION (see Respiratory Patterns in Part 3, Pulmonary System)**

⬤ **CHIARI MALFORMATIONS**

These are a group of abnormalities of the craniocervical junction characterized by the hindbrain descending down through the foramen magnum. The malformation is divided into three types:

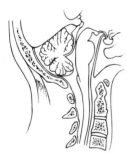 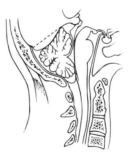 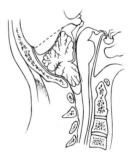

| Type I. Descent of cerebellar tonsils through foramen magnum. | Type II. Marked descent of hindbrain structures (pons, medulla, and fourth ventricle) through foramen magnum. Often associated with myelomeningocoele. | Type III. Hindbrain herniation into a high cervical meningocoele. |

FIGURE 1-10 Chiari malformation. (Reprinted with permission. Palmer, J. [1996]. *Manual of neurosurgery.* New York: Churchill Livingstone.)

(*continued*)

The abnormality is rare, affecting only 1 in 10,000 to 15,000, with males more commonly affected than females. Average age for diagnosis is estimated at 30 to 40 years for adults and 11 years for children. There is a wide variance as to how these patients present clinically, probably accounting for frequent delays in diagnosis. Most patients require surgical intervention, which affords no cure but rather relief of shunting of CSF in the presence of hydrocephalus, decompression of a hindbrain hernia, or drainage of any hydromyelic cavity.

CHOROID PLEXUS

The choroid plexus is a special capillary bed that filters blood, so that as the blood passes through it, it comes out cerebrospinal fluid.

CHVOSTEK'S SIGN (see also Trousseau's Sign)

Chvostek's sign is a twitch of facial muscles, upper lip, and eye following sharp tap to facial nerve (seventh cranial nerve) anterior to the ear, just below the temple. It is related to a decreased serum calcium level.

CIRCLE OF WILLIS

The circle of Willis is an anatomical juncture representing an anastomosis of four major vessels: posterior cerebral, anterior cerebral, internal carotid, and posterior/anterior communicating. The "circle" is the most common site for an intracranial aneurysm.

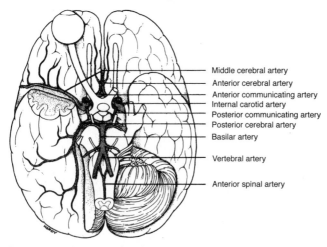

Middle cerebral artery
Anterior cerebral artery
Anterior communicating artery
Internal carotid artery
Posterior communicating artery
Posterior cerebral artery
Basilar artery
Vertebral artery
Anterior spinal artery

FIGURE 1-11 The circle of Willis seen from below the brain.

(*continued*)

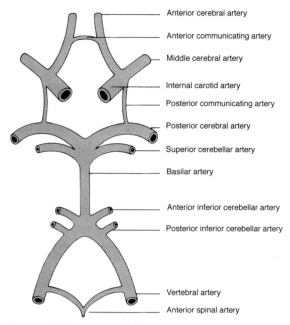

FIGURE 1-12 The circle of Willis.

● CLUSTER BREATHING (see Respiratory Patterns in Part 3, Pulmonary System)

● COMA (see also Caloric Test)

Coma is a state defined as being unconscious, unarousable, and unresponsive to touch or sound. Coma is caused by one of two things:

1. Damage to both cerebral hemispheres
2. Damage to ascending reticular activating system in brain stem

The caloric test differentiates between the two (see Caloric Test).

● CONSENSUAL REFLEX

A normal reflex, the consensual reflex is demonstrated by constriction of opposite pupil when light stimulates one eye.

REMEMBER: **Consensus = both agree.**

CORNEAL REFLEX

The corneal reflex tests the fifth cranial nerve, the trigeminal. Touch cornea with wisp of cotton and observe for blink reflex, or apply pressure to supraorbital ridge and observe for facial grimacing (reflex is decreased or absent on same side as hemiplegia).

CRANIAL NERVES

The 12 pairs of symmetrically arranged cranial nerves are attached to the brain and exit through a foramen at its base. The site where the fibers composing the nerve enter or leave the brain surface is usually termed the *superficial origin* of the nerve; the more deeply placed group of cells from which the fibers arise or around which they terminate is called the *nucleus of origin*.

To remember the names of the 12 nerves, remember the mnemonic "On old Olympian towering tops, a Fin and German viewed some hops." **But,** because so many of the nerves begin with the same letter, also remember the mnemonic "Little people can only imitate big champions." This gives the second letter (or third, if both second letters are the same) of the nerve. To remember the type of nerve, remember the mnemonic "Some say marry money, but my brother says (it is) bad business marrying money" (s = sensory; m = motor; b = both sensory and motor).

(continued)

NOTES

TABLE 1-1. Cranial Nerves

Mnemonic		Cranial Nerves and Function	Type
First Letter	*Underlined Letter*		
On	(little)	I **Olfactory.** Smells	S (some)
Old	(people)	II **Optic.** Sees; Snellen Chart	S (say)
Olympian	(can)	III **Oculomotor.** Moves eyes, with 4 and 6. Constricts pupils, accommodates.	M (marry)

REMEMBER: CN III = pillars. Opens eyes.

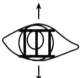

Towering	(only)	IV **Trochlear.** Moves eyes, with 3 and 6. Downward, inward.	M (money)
Tops	(imitate)	V **Trigeminal.** Sensations from face, cornea, teeth, tongue, nasal, oral mucosa. Chews (see also corneal reflex).	B (but)
A	(big)	VI **Abducens.** Moves eyes, with 3 and 4. Laterally.	M (my)
Fin		VII **Facial.** Moves eyes, salivation, taste (anterior 2/3 of tongue).	B (brother)

REMEMBER: CN VII = a hook. Closes eyes.

And	(champions)	VIII **Acoustic.** Hears. Regulates balance (see also Caloric Test, Rinne Test, Weber Test).	S (says) (it is)
German		IX **Glossopharyngeal.** Taste (posterior 1/3 of tongue), swallow, gag, pharyngeal sensation, salivation. Reflex control of BP, pulse, respirations.	B (bad)
Viewed		X **Vagus.** Sensation and movement of pharynx, larynx, thoracic and abdominal viscera.	B (business)
Some		XI **Spinal Accessory.** Turns head, lifts shoulders.	M (marrying)
Hops		XII **Hypoglossal.** Moves tongue.	M (money)

○ CRANIAL NERVE EXAM

TABLE 1-2. Cranial Nerve Assessment

Cranial Nerve	Assessment	Comments
I Olfactory	**Sense of smell** Usually deferred	Deficits noted in only a few cases, usually with lesion in the parasellar area
II Optic	**Vision** Monitor while working with patient; observe for difficulty with ADLs Ask patient to identify how many fingers are being held up or to read menu or newspaper Use Rosenbaum Pocket Vision Screener to assess vision in each eye Monitor for visual field cuts by checking upper and lower quadrants while patient focuses on your nose	Common deficits; deficits can cause blindness in one eye, bitemporal hemianopia, or homonymous hemianopia
III Oculomotor	**Pupil constriction; elevation of upper eyelid** Assess size, shape, and direct light reaction of pupils	Changes are common with a number of progressing neurological problems
III Oculomotor IV Trochlear VI Abducent	**Extraocular movement** Tested together in conscious, cooperative patient; ask patient to follow a pencil tip through the six cardinal eye movements	Deficits are common; inability to move the eyes in one or more directions; or strabismus
V Trigeminal	**Sensation to face; mastication muscles** Often deferred If assessed, patient must be cooperative and able to accurately report facial sensation to stimulation **Afferent limb of corneal reflex**	Deficits found in trigeminal neuralgia and sometimes with acoustic neuroma Corneal reflex assessed in trigeminal neuralgia; can assess reflex in unconscious patient
VII Facial	**Muscles for facial expression; efferent limb of corneal reflex** In cooperative patient, ask him or her to smile, show teeth, puff cheeks, wrinkle brow; observe for symmetry of face In a comatose patient, tickle each nasal passage, one at a time, by inserting a cotton-tipped applicator; observe for facial movement	Total unilateral facial weakness, called Bell's palsy Unilateral from below the eye and down, seen in stroke Note the difference between central and peripheral facial involvement
VIII Acoustic	**Hearing and balance** Usually deferred May note deficit while working with patient	Deficits with acoustic neuroma, cerebellopontine angle tumors, Meniere's disease
IX Glossopharyngeal X Vagus	**Palate, pharynx, vocal cords, and gag reflex;** tested together because of overlap In conscious patient, have patient open mouth and say "ah," assess gag reflex In unconscious patient, assess gag reflex	Deficits common in posterior fossa lesions Gag reflex is a brain stem reflex and has prognostic value in unconscious patient

(continued)

TABLE 1-2. Cranial Nerve Assessment (Continued)

XI Spinal accessory	**Shrug shoulders and move head side to side** Usually deferred	Deficits common in posterior fossa lesions
XII Hypoglossal	**Movement of tongue** In conscious patient, ask him or her to stick out the tongue	Deficits common in posterior fossa lesions

Note: This table summarizes **assessment at the bedside**. Although a baseline assessment of all cranial nerves is recommended, this may not always be possible. In addition, whereas frequent assessment of particular cranial nerves is critical in certain conditions, it may be safely deferred in other conditions.

⬛ CRANIOPHARYNGIOMA (see Tumors, Neurogenic)

⬛ CREUTZFELDT-JAKOB DISEASE

Creutzfeldt-Jakob disease (CJD) is a degenerative neurologic disease that is rapid and fatal, similar to "mad cow" disease (bovine spongiform encephalopathy, or BSE). Though the two are similar, no correlation of a relationship between them is evident. Onset of CJD manifests itself as confusion, then it progresses rapidly to coma and death, usually within 2 years, often within 1 year. The disorder is seen in adults with an average age of 60 years. Because it is infectious, standard precautions should be taken with invasive procedures or contaminated body fluids, especially spinal fluid or brain tissue.

TABLE 1-3. Infectivity of Tissues, Body Fluids, and Excretions from Patients with CJD

Tissue, Fluids, or Excreta Containing Infectious Agent				
Consistently *(>50% of attempts)*	*Sometimes* *(4–50% of attempts)*	*Occasionally**	*Never†*	
Brain	CSF	Blood	Adrenal	Nasal mucus
Spinal Cord	Kidney	Urine	Feces	Nerve
Eye	Liver		Heart	Saliva
	Lung		Marrow	Sputum
	Lymph node		Muscle	Tears
	Spleen			

*Transmission of CJD from blood and urine of patients to animals was not confirmed in our laboratory (blood or blood components, 12 attempts; urine, 11 attempts).
  †Three or more attempts were negative. A smaller number of attempts were also negative for intestine, thyroid, fat, gingiva, prostate, testis, placenta or amnion, semen, vaginal secretions, and breast milk.
  Asher, D.M. (1995). Spongiform encephalopathies. In *Manual of Clinical Microbiology*, 6th ed. Washington, DC: American Society of Microbiology.

⬤ CSF (see Cerebrospinal Fluid)

⬤ CUSHING'S REFLEX (see also Cushing's Triad)

Cushing's reflex causes the symptoms of Cushing's triad (see Cushing's Triad). When CSF pressure and the pressure within the intracranial cerebral arteries starts to equilibrate, the cerebral arteries become compressed and begin to collapse. This compromises cerebral blood flow. Cushing's reflex is activated, and the arterial pressure rises to a level higher than the CSF pressure, allowing cerebral blood flow to be reestablished and ischemia to be relieved. The blood pressure is maintained at a new, higher level, and the brain is protected from further loss of adequate blood flow.

⬤ CUSHING'S TRIAD (see also Cushing's Reflex)

The triad refers to three signs caused by Cushing's reflex:

1. Bradycardia
2. Hypertension
3. Bradypnea (often irregular)

It is indicative of an advanced increase in intracranial pressure, that is, the brain's "last gasp." The triad and the reflex are late findings, and irreversible neurologic damage may have already occurred by the time they are recognized.

⬤ DECEREBRATE

Decerebration is demonstrated by extension of involved extremities with outward pronation of the wrists and hands. Legs are stiffly extended at the knees with the feet plantar flexed. This indicates disruption of motor fibers in the midbrain and brain stem. *REMEMBER:* "Without cerebrum" or "extension."

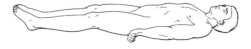

Figure 1-13 Decerebrate posturing.

⬤ DECORTICATE

Decortication is demonstrated by flexion of the upper extremities and extension and internal rotation of the lower extremities on the side of the lesion. It is seen in patients with interruption of cortical nerve fibers, but intact pathways through the brain stem. *REMEMBER:* "To the core" or "without cortex."

(continued)

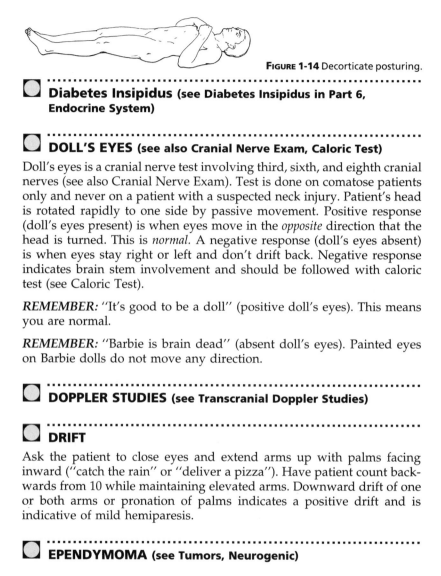

FIGURE 1-14 Decorticate posturing.

Diabetes Insipidus (see Diabetes Insipidus in Part 6, Endocrine System)

DOLL'S EYES (see also Cranial Nerve Exam, Caloric Test)

Doll's eyes is a cranial nerve test involving third, sixth, and eighth cranial nerves (see also Cranial Nerve Exam). Test is done on comatose patients only and never on a patient with a suspected neck injury. Patient's head is rotated rapidly to one side by passive movement. Positive response (doll's eyes present) is when eyes move in the *opposite* direction that the head is turned. This is *normal*. A negative response (doll's eyes absent) is when eyes stay right or left and don't drift back. Negative response indicates brain stem involvement and should be followed with caloric test (see Caloric Test).

REMEMBER: "It's good to be a doll" (positive doll's eyes). This means you are normal.

REMEMBER: "Barbie is brain dead" (absent doll's eyes). Painted eyes on Barbie dolls do not move any direction.

DOPPLER STUDIES (see Transcranial Doppler Studies)

DRIFT

Ask the patient to close eyes and extend arms up with palms facing inward ("catch the rain" or "deliver a pizza"). Have patient count backwards from 10 while maintaining elevated arms. Downward drift of one or both arms or pronation of palms indicates a positive drift and is indicative of mild hemiparesis.

EPENDYMOMA (see Tumors, Neurogenic)

EPIDURAL ANALGESIA

Epidural catheter is placed in the "potential" space along the spinal column, located between the dura mater and the ligamentum flavum. The catheter may be placed in the lumbar or thoracic spine, but L1 to L5 is most common. It provides excellent pain relief without affecting motor function and without diminishing the sensations of touch, temperature, and proprioception.

(continued)

Opiates are injected into the epidural space and bind to fat. Fat carries the opiates across the dura mater into the subarachnoid space and binds to opiate receptors in the spinal cord. Transmission of pain impulses is thus inhibited.

TABLE 1-4. Common Epidural Medications

	Fentanyl	Hydromorphone (Dilaudid)	Morphine
DOSE:	50–100 μg	0.5–2 mg	5–10 mg
ONSET:	4–10 min	13 min	23 min
RELIEF:	20 min	25 min	45 min
DURATION:	4–5 hr	1–12 hr	12–18 hr
SOLUBLE:	High lipid solubility = binds quickly to fat = rapid onset	Moderate	Low lipid solubility (water soluble) = less rapid binding, slower onset, and longer duration; also has greater potential for side effects

Administration of Analgesia:

Note: Many institutions require personnel to be certified before being allowed to administer drugs epidurally.

1. Draw up (filtered needle) ordered amount of preservative-free opiate and preservative-free normal saline in 10-cc syringe.

2. Using empty 3-cc syringe, assess placement of catheter by slowly aspirating for 30 seconds. More than 1 cc of fluid indicates intrathecal placement. Presence of blood indicates vascular placement. **Terminate** procedure.

3. If no aspirate, or aspirate <1 cc, administer medication, maintaining sterility of cap.

Note: If injection is difficult, reposition the patient supine with spine flexed. This increases the intervertebral space and decreases compression on the catheter.

4. Monitor and record BP and pulse at least every 30 minutes × 2 hr. Patient should be on continuous pulse oximeter.

REMEMBER: **Never** use alcohol swabs, because alcohol (which acts as a preservative) is toxic to the spinal cord. And **always** use preservative-free solutions.

⬤ EPIDURAL HEMATOMA (see also Herniation)

Epidural hematoma is usually related to trauma, brain stem contusion, or basilar or temporal bone fracture. It is caused by mass influx of blood into the epidural space. Signs are *rapid* onset of decreased LOC, ipsilateral (same side) fixed pupil, and increased intracranial pressure. Watch for uncal herniation (see Herniation). Epidural hematoma is treated by surgical evacuation. A lumbar puncture is contraindicated in an expanding lesion as it can cause herniation and it is usually inaccurate (CSF needs to flow freely to be accurate).

⬤ EPILEPSY (see Seizures)

⬤ FORAMEN MAGNUM

Foramen magnum means "large hole" and is the point at which brain stem becomes spinal cord.

⬤ GLASGOW COMA SCALE

Scoring of eye opening:

- 4 Opens eyes spontaneously when the nurse approaches
- 3 Opens eyes in response to speech (normal or shout)
- 2 Opens eyes only to painful stimuli (eg, squeezing of nail beds)
- 1 Does not open eyes to painful stimuli

Scoring of best motor response:

- 6 Can obey a simple command, such as "Lift your left hand off the bed"
- 5 Localizes to painful stimuli and attempts to remove source
- 4 Purposeless movement in response to pain
- 3 Flexes elbows and wrists while extending lower legs to pain
- 2 Extends upper and lower extremities to pain
- 1 No motor response to pain on any limb

(continued)

Scoring of best verbal response:
- 5 Oriented to time, place, and person
- 4 Converses, although confused
- 3 Speaks only in words or phrases that make little or no sense
- 2 Responds with incomprehensible sounds (eg, groans)
- 1 No verbal response

(From Hickey, J.V. (1997). *Clinical practice of Neurological and Neurosurgical Nursing,* 4th ed. Philadelphia: Lippincott-Raven.)

GLIOBLASTOMA (see Tumors, Neurogenic)

GLIOMA (see Tumors, Neurogenic)

GLYCOLYSIS

Glycolysis provides energy in the form of ATP by anaerobically metabolizing glucose. Glucose is a "cheap" source of ATP for the brain. Therefore, during hypoxia, the rate of glucose breakdown (glycolysis) is increased. Remember, the brain does **not** need insulin to use glucose; a constant supply of both O_2 and glucose is what it needs for metabolism. Because the brain has no glucose store, it therefore depends on a constant blood supply.

GUILLAIN-BARRÉ SYNDROME

The demyelination of lower motor neurons of this syndrome affects spinal and cranial nerves (peripheral nervous system). Guillain-Barré syndrome is also known as infectious polyneuritis. It is an ascending paralysis and is usually symmetrical, with no alteration of consciousness. It may occur after a viral infection, usually of the upper respiratory tract. The most serious complication is respiratory arrest (decreased work ability of diaphragm and breathing muscles). Signs are decreased vital capacity and increased protein in CSF. UTIs are a common complication.

HALO SIGN (see also Cerebrospinal Fluid)

The patient with a CSF leak may experience otorrhea (leakage of CSF from the ear), rhinorrhea (leakage of CSF from the nares), leaking of CSF into the nasopharynx, or CSF fluid collection or drainage at an operative site. CSF drainage can sometimes be identified by a characteristic "halo" sign, or a yellowish ring surrounding the drainage on dressings or linens.

(continued)

To differentiate between mucous and a CSF leak, the drainage can be tested with a glucose-indicator strip (Dextrostix). If CSF is present, the indicator has a positive reaction, because CSF contains sugar.

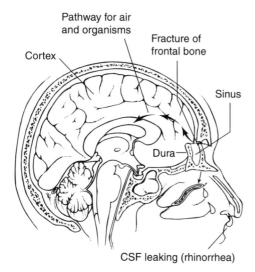

Pathway for air and organisms

Fracture of frontal bone

Cortex

Sinus

Dura

CSF leaking (rhinorrhea)

FIGURE 1-15 CSF leak.

⬤ HERNIATION

Neurologically, herniation is divided into three types:

1. Central (transtentorial) herniation is evidenced by compression and downward displacement of the hemispheres, resulting in compression against the tentorium cerebelli. Signs include small pupils (1–3 mm) at first, then both pupils dilate. It is usually seen in chronic disorders.

2. Uncal herniation is a displacement of the temporal lobe (uncus) against the brain stem and third cranial nerve. It is found in CVA with ipsilateral pupil dilation. It is also seen in neurologic emergencies, such as epidural hematoma. Patient exhibits a "blown" pupil, because the herniation compresses the cranial nerves.

3. Infratentorial herniation is a compression on the brain stem or cerebellum, either upward against the tentorium cerebelli or downward through the foramen magnum.

(*continued*)

TABLE 1-5. Types of Herniation*

Central (Transtentorial)

	Early	Late
Pupils	Small, reactive bilaterally	Bilateral fixed, dilated
Level of arousal	Difficulty with concentration; agitated or drowsy	Stupor leads to coma
Motor	Contralateral hemiparesis	Bilateral decortication, decerebration, flacidity
Respiration	Pauses, central neurogenic hyperventilation	Cheyne-Stokes, ataxia
Extraocular signs	Normal or slightly roving	Dysconjugate gaze, extraocular paralysis

Uncal (Lateral Transtentorial)

	Early	Late
Pupils	Unilateral dilated pupil; sluggish nonreactive	Dilated and fixed
Level of arousal	Normal to restless	Stupor may rapidly become coma
Motor	Slight weakness, pronator drift	Decortication, decerebration, flaccidity
Respiration	Normal	Cheyne-Stokes, ataxia, respiratory arrest
Extraocular signs	Ptosis	Extraocular paralysis

Infratentorial

	Early	Late
Pupils	Midposition or small and nonreactive	Bilateral fixed
Level of arousal	Stupor	Coma
Motor	Hemiparesis, hemiplegia	Decortication, decerebration, flaccidity
Respiration	Variable depending on level of lesion	Respiratory arrest
Extraocular signs	Ophthalmoplegias; early loss of upward gaze	Extraocular paralysis

*An important point to keep in mind when observing a patient with a possible herniation is that there is a predicatable order to the development of the signs and symptoms. The neurologic deterioration in both central and uncal hernation proceeds in an orderly scheme (the diencephalon, midbrain, pons, and finally medulla are effected by increasing pressure). Notice the last stages of central and uncal herniation are the same.
Revised and adapted from Hickey, J.V. (1997). *The Clinical Practice of Neurological and Neurosurgical Nursing,* 4th ed. Philadelphia: Lippincott-Raven.

HOMONYMOUS HEMIANOPIA

Homonymous hemianopia is the loss of vision in half the field of each eye (hemi- = half, anopia = of each field). It indicates damage to the optic nerve.

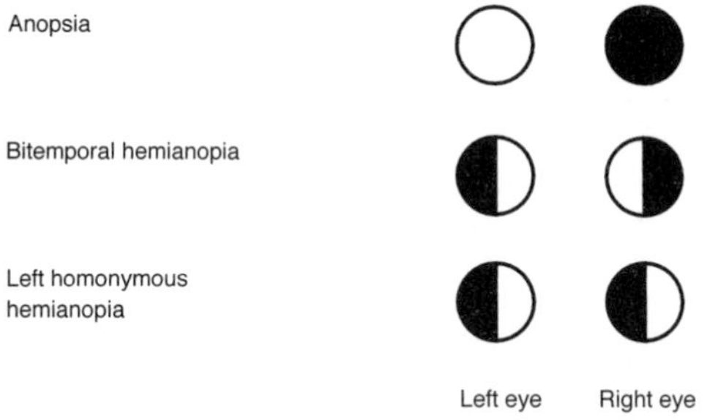

Anopsia

Bitemporal hemianopia

Left homonymous
hemianopia

Left eye   Right eye

FIGURE 1-16 Visual field defects. *Black area* = no vision.

HUNT AND HESS SCALE (see Aneurysms)

HYDROCEPHALUS

Hydrocephalus is an abnormal accumulation of CSF in the cranial vault. In infants, head enlarges. In adults, because the cranium is fixed in size and cannot give, there is no enlargement. The mounting pressure caused by the excess fluid squeezes the brain tissue against the skull, causing tissue atrophy and tissue death, as well as seizures. Hydrocephalus can be surgically corrected by placing a ventroperitoneal shunt (VP shunt) that runs from the brain ventricle, under the skin, downward to the peritoneum for drainage.

INCREASED INTRACRANIAL PRESSURE (see also Cerebral Perfusion Pressure, Cushing's Reflex, Cushing's Triad, Intracranial Pressure Monitoring, Monro-Kellie Hypothesis)

When the nondistendable intracranial cavity is filled to capacity with noncompressible contents, that is, CSF, blood, or brain tissue, the result is an increase in intracranial pressure, or ICP.

Normal ICP	3–15 mmHg
Severe increase	>20 mmHg

(continued)

Conditions causing an increase in ICP:

Increased brain volume	• Space-occupying lesions such as epidural and subdural hematomas, abscesses, or aneurysms. • Cerebral edema related to head injuries, cardiopulmonary arrest, and metabolic encephalopathies

Increased blood volume	• Obstruction of venous outflow
	• Hyperemia
	• Hypercapnia
	    Remember this key point:
	    Receptors in the brain constantly analyze blood gases. Therefore an **increase** in PCO_2 (hypoventilation) means **vasodilation** of cerebral vessels and an **increase** in blood flow to the brain: **ICP rises.** Conversely, a **decrease** in PCO_2 (hyperventilation) means **vasoconstriction** of cerebral vessels and a **decrease** of blood flow to the brain: **ICP decreases.**
	• Disease states associated with increased blood volume
	• Reye's syndrome

Increased CSF	• Increased production of CSF • Decreased absorption of CSF • Obstruction of CSF flow

(continued)

NOTES

Factors contributing to increased ICP:

Hypercapnia ($PCO_2 > 45$ mmHg)	• Sleep, sedation, shallow respirations, coma, neuromuscular impairment, improper mechanical ventilator settings
Hypoxemia ($PCO_2 < 30$ mmHg)	• Insufficient oxygen concentration in supplemental oxygen therapy; inadequate lung perfusion; inadequate lung ventilation; drug-induced cerebral vasodilation; administration of nicotinic acid, Cyclandelate, histamine, and anesthetic agents such as halothane, enflurane, isoflurane, and nitrous oxide
Valsalva's maneuver	• Straining at stool, moving or turning in bed, coughing, sneezing
Body positioning	• Any position that obstructs venous return from the brain, ie, Trendelenburg's, prone, extreme flexion of hips, neck flexion
Isometric muscle contractions	• Isometric exercises, ie, pushing against resistance, shivering, decerebration
REM sleep	• Rapid eye movements are associated with cerebral activity; sleep arousal also increases ICP
Noxious stimuli	• Visceral discomfort, painful procedures, stimuli associated with assessment, loud noises

Classic signs and symptoms of increased ICP:

Decreased LOC	• Confusion, increasing headache, blurred vision, vomiting
Impaired motor function	• Change in motor ability, change in cranial nerve function (especially oculomotor function)
Alteration in pupil reflex	• Papilledema (edema of the optic disc; a positive sign of increased ICP but not seen in acute intracranial hypertension), sluggish or absent light responses, photophobia
Change in vital signs	• A change in baseline from one assessment to the next may indicate a change in neurologic status

(continued)

Management of increased ICP (>15 mmHg = one or several of the following):

Hyperventilate	• Keep PCO$_2$ at 25–30 mmHg, no less than 25 mmHg. Causes vasoconstriction, thus decreasing cerebral blood volume and decreasing ICP.
Osmotic diuretics	• Urea, mannitol, glycerol decrease interstitial fluid in brain.
CSF drainage	• Drain CSF via intraventricular cannulas or subarachnoid screws.
Barbituates	• Phenobarbital or pentobarbital produces complete unresponsiveness and therefore decreases metabolic demands. **Note:** Patient must be intubated and ventilated with continuous arterial blood pressure monitoring.
Hypothermia	• Decreases metabolic demand.
Hypovolemia	• Deliver only hypertonic or isotonic fluids, **no D5W or 1/2NS.** Fluid would go from blood vessels to brain matter and increase edema.
Steroids	• (dexamethasone, methylprednisolone) Action is unclear, but steroids may stabilize cell membrane and slow leaking of fluid into brain. • Does not apply to trauma.

INTRACRANIAL PRESSURE MONITORING (see also Cerebral Perfusion Pressure, Increased Intracranial Pressure)

- **The waveform:** The ICP waveform results from transmission of arterial and venous pressure waves through the CSF and brain parenchyma.

Normal ICP	3–15 mmHg
Severe increase	>20 mmHg

(*continued*)

NOTES

The normal ICP waveform has an upstroke that corresponds to systole and three small peaks of decreasing amplitude. The waveform resembles a somewhat dampened arterial waveform.

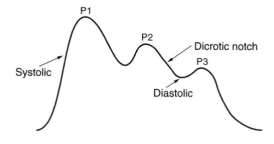

Figure **1-17** Normal ICP waveform. (Adapted from Hudak, C.M., Gallo, B.M., & Morton, P.G. [1998]. Critical care nursing [7th ed.]. Philadelphia: Lippincott-Raven.)

A waves (plateau waves) are seen in the decompensatory stage of increased ICP and are associated with cerebral ischemia. They may last 2 to 20 minutes and occur from a baseline of an already increased ICP (usually >20 mmHg, but may be as high as 40–50 mmHg). Physician should be notified.

B waves (sawtooth waves) occur in multiples and are associated with fluctuations of ICP related to respiratory patterns. They may occur every 30 seconds to 2 minutes with an ICP in the range of 20 to 50 mmHg. They signify a decreased intracranial compliance and are a precursor of A waves.

C waves (small, rhythmic waves) occur four to eight times per minute. They correlate to normal fluctuations in respiration and blood pressure. They have no clinical significance but may be associated with increased ICP by as much as 20 mmHg.

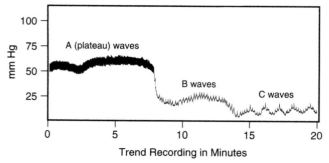

Figure **1-18** Intracranial pressure waves. Composite drawing of A (plateau) waves, B waves, and C waves.

(*continued*)

The monitoring devices:

VENTRICULOSTOMY

The ventriculostomy is considered the "gold standard" for ICP monitoring. Though its accuracy is unquestionable, the problem lies in the fact that it is associated with the highest risk of infection and requires that the user have a sound working knowledge of the system. The ventriculostomy is inserted into the anterior horn of the lateral ventricle (sometimes posterior horn), usually in the nondominant hemisphere, and can be incorporated into a hydraulic, fluid-filled, or fiberoptic monitoring system.

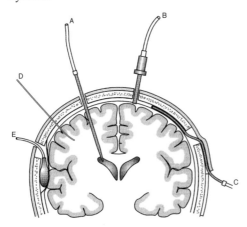

FIGURE 1-19 Intracranial pressure (ICP) monitoring systems. **(A)** intraventricular; **(B)** subarachnoid; **(C)** subdural; **(D)** parenchymal; **(E)** epidural.

SETUP SPECIFICS

Head of bed should be elevated 20° to 30°.

If a fluid-filled transduced system, prime line with nonbacteriostatic normal saline. **No air bubbles** in system.

Level transducer at the foramen of Monro (halfway between the outer canthus of the eye and the tragus of the ear). Remember to relevel with any change in the patient's position.

Connect to bedside monitor and zero the monitor (open to air, closed to the patient). Remember to rezero with any change in the patient's position. Check for adequate waveform.

MD may order the drainage collection chamber to be elevated at a specific level above the patient for CSF drainage. This is usually in cm H_2O, but it can also be in mmHg. These are different levels, so be sure to be consistent with the order. Alternately, orders may be received to drain a specific amount of CSF, then clamp the ventriculostomy, or to open the ventriculostomy to drainage when a certain ICP level is reached.

(continued)

If the patient's ICP exceeds the level at which the bag is positioned, CSF should flow into the bag. Conversely, if the bag is leveled too low, the patient drains CSF that should not be drained. This is a dangerous situation.

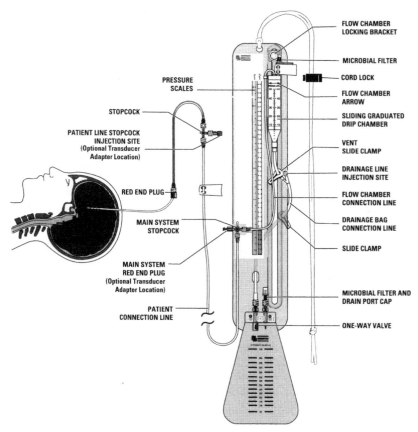

FIGURE 1-20 Becker external drainage and monitoring system for intracranial pressure monitoring and intermittent cerebrospinal fluid drainage. (Courtesy of Medtronic PS Medical, Goleta, CA.)

Be sure all tubing is **air-bubble-free** and **never** fast-flush the ventricular catheter.

To obtain CSF samples, always use the port **below** the collection chamber, and swab with **Betadine only.**

Remember to always close the stopcock to the patient during temporary change of position, for example, for X-ray films or turning, and remember to always reopen it on completion of task.

(*continued*)

TROUBLESHOOTING: FLUID-FILLED SYSTEM

Loss of waveform	Check stopcock connections
	Check for air in system
	Check monitor cable
	Increase gain or range on monitor
False high or low	Rezero and calibrate
	Reposition transducer
	Check system for air bubbles
Low ICP pressure	Check patient for otorrhea and rhinorrhea

FIBEROPTICS

The fiberoptic catheter is extremely versatile and can be placed in virtually any intracranial location because the transducer is at the tip of the catheter. Usually, it is incorporated within a subarachnoid bolt or ventriculostomy. The system requires no flush and is calibrated only once immediately prior to insertion. The problems of a fluid-filled system are eliminated, but the system is difficult to maintain securely fixed to the patient, and the fragile fiberoptic filaments are easily damaged as a result of tension or catheter crimping, all too often rendering the system inoperative.

TROUBLESHOOTING: FIBEROPTIC SYSTEM

Loss of waveform	Check cable connections, reconnect as needed
	Increase gain or range
	Assist physician in repositioning catheter
False high or low	Assist physician in repositioning catheter
Monitor reads 888	Assist physician in repositioning catheter
Microprocessor and bedside	Rezero and calibrate
monitor do not correlate	Check connections

SUBARACHNOID BOLT

There is no penetration of the brain necessary for insertion of this device, because it is "screwed" into the subarachnoid space. The risk of infection is markedly decreased. However, the system affords no way to drain CSF and is unreliable at high ICP pressures, when the brain tissue herniates up into the monitoring device.

(continued)

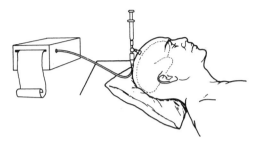

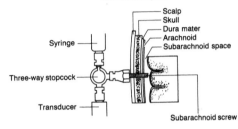

Close-up of placement into
subarachnoid space

Scalp
Skull
Dura mater
Arachnoid
Subarachnoid space

Syringe

Three-way stopcock

Transducer

Subarachnoid screw

FIGURE 1-21 Subarachnoid bolt.

TROUBLESHOOTING: SUBARACHNOID BOLT

Loss of waveform	Check connections
	Check for air in system
	Check monitor cable
	Increase gain or range
False high or low	Recalibrate
	Check system for air bubbles
Low ICP pressure	Check patient for otorrhea and rhinorrhea

KERNIG'S SIGN (see also Brudzinski's Sign)

To test for Kernig's sign, flex patient's hip 90°, extend knee. Response is positive if there is pain and/or spasm and indicates a bleed into subarachnoid space. It is also positive in meningitis.

KUSSMAUL'S RESPIRATION (See Respiratory Patterns in Part 3, Pulmonary System)

◎ LOBE FUNCTIONS

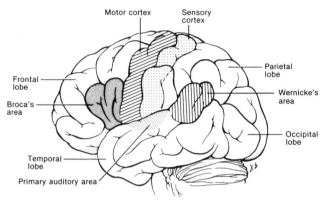

FIGURE 1-22 Cerebrocortical areas involved in communication.

FRONTAL	Plan for future. Speech.
	Prefrontal: Controls respiration, GI activity, circulation, pupillary reactions, emotions. Helps regulate personality, thought processes, intellect, math ability, and concentration.
	Broca's area: Controls ability to articulate speech. Contained in one hemisphere and is almost always dominant in the left. Damage to this area may cause motor aphasia.
	Written speech area: Controls ability to write words. Does not matter if right or left handed, this area is usually situated in the left cerebral hemisphere.
TEMPORAL	Second weakest bone in skull. Deals with sound.
	Wernicke's area: Works to understand spoken word and written language.
	Auditory speech: Integrates sound into pitch, quality, loudness.
	Postcranial area: Controls body's sensory areas.
OCCIPITAL	Visual.
	Visual sensory area: Integrates visual stimulation for size, form, motion, color.
CEREBELLUM	Divided into two hemispheres, each composed of gray and white matter. Governs walking, balance, coordination, and muscular memory.
	REMEMBER: A lesion in the cerebellum presents signs and symptoms (eg, ataxia) on the **same side** of the body (the **ipsilateral** side).

◯ LUMBAR PUNCTURE (see also Cerebrospinal Fluid; Lab Values: CSF Fluid in Part 10, Labs; Spinal Cord)

Lumbar puncture is performed below the second lumbar vertebra so spinal cord won't be hit. It is diagnostic for subarachnoid hemorrhage and meningitis.

| Normal lumbar pressures: 8 to 180 cm H_2O with patient side lying
| Via ICP monitoring: 4 to 15 mmHg

Procedure is contraindicated with advanced signs of increased intracranial pressure.

◯ MEAN ARTERIAL PRESSURE (see also Increased Intracranial Pressure)

$$\frac{\text{Systolic blood pressure} + (\text{diastolic blood pressure} \times 2)}{3} \qquad REMEMBER: \frac{1 + 2}{3}$$

| Normal: 70 to 110 mmHg

◯ MEDULLOBLASTOMA (see Tumors, Neurogenic)

◯ MENINGIOMA (see Tumors, Neurogenic)

◯ MENINGITIS (see also Brudzinski's Sign, Cranial Nerves, Kernig's Sign, Lumbar Puncture)

Diagnosis of meningitis is related to pathologic organism found in subarachnoid space (meninges) causing disruption of the blood-brain barrier. Exudate forms and collects, resulting in congestion of tissue, edema, and increased ICP. Meningitis leads to necrosis of the cortex and nerve damage. Several sources are possible: sinus, midear, skull fracture, drains, and so on. Pay attention to eighth cranial nerve (acoustic) because disease itself can cause deafness. Cause may be bacterial or viral.

The signs and symptoms form a common triad: stiff neck, fever, acute onset of altered neurologic status. Signs may also include headache, positive Kernig's and Brudzinski's sign, increased ICP, and petechiae. The two types of meningitis, bacterial and viral, are diagnosed by lumbar puncture, in which the CSF may exhibit the following (dependent on the organism):

1. Cloudy, turbid color
2. Increase in protein (higher in bacterial than viral)
3. Decrease in glucose (usually in bacterial; may be normal in viral)

(continued)

REMEMBER: **Bacteria like to eat things and viruses don't.** Therefore, in bacterial meningitis, the bacteria "gobble up" all the glucose (it's so yummy and sweet!), resulting in **decreased glucose** in the CSF and **increased protein** because it's leftover.

Also, in differentiating bacterial from viral meningitis, remember there are increased WBCs in the CSF (>1200), the polymorphs are elevated, and there are no lymphocytes in the bacterial form.

Bacterial meningitis is treated with large doses of penicillin, and isolation of patient is required. The disease is further broken down into three subtypes:

Haemophilus influenzae (in children)	Gram − *Haemophilus influenzae*
Meningococcal (young adult)	Gram − *Neisseria meningitidis*
Pneumococcal (after 40)	Gram + *Streptococcus pneumoniae*

Viral meningitis is also known as acute benign lymphocytic meningitis or acute aseptic meningitis. It is related to an enterovirus, but isolation is **not** necessary. It is usually seen in children, and complete recovery is standard.

 MONRO-KELLIE HYPOTHESIS (see also Increased Intracranial Pressure)

The skull is a closed box containing three intracranial volumes:

1. CSF (about 10%)

2. Intravascular blood (about 10%)

3. Brain tissue (about 80%)

An increase in any one of the three, without a decrease in one or both of the others, will result in an increase in ICP.

 MULTIPLE SCLEROSIS

MS is a chronic, progressive demyelinating disease of the nervous system with an overgrowth of glial cells in the white substance of the brain and spinal cord. Early in the disease, the lesions formed by the destruction of the myelin sheath are temporary; later, they are permanent. Some common symptoms are:

• Blurred vision

• Diplopia

• Nystagmus

(continued)

- Weakness, tingling of extremity
- Ataxia
- Paralysis (usually of lower extremities)
- Intention tremor

These symptoms often appear gradually then disappear, only to return later in months or even years. Some patients have severe, long-lasting exacerbations, whereas others experience only occasional, mild symptoms for several years after onset. The course is unknown, and there is no cure.

 MUSCULAR DYSTROPHY

Muscular dystrophy is characterized by progressive weakness and final atrophy of groups of muscles. The cause is unknown. It develops mostly in children, and in at least half of all cases, there is a history of at least one other family member who had the disease. There are several forms, pseudohypertrophic being one of the most common. It is characterized by enlargement of the calf muscles, accompanied by limitation of muscle function. There is no effective medical treatment known. The disease does not have remissions and gets progressively worse. Few affected children live to adulthood.

 MYASTHENIA GRAVIS

Myasthenia gravis is a disease of the neuromuscular junction character-ized by abnormal muscle fatigue brought on by activity and improving with rest. The etiology is unknown, though a link to autoimmunity is suspected. Sometimes, removal of the thymus is helpful. Diagnosis is based on the Tensilon (edrophonium) test. Tensilon is a rapid-acting anticholinesterase and causes the symptoms of the disease to rapidly and transiently improve.

A myasthenia crisis occurs when there is not enough cholinesterase in the system, or when a tolerance for it has been reached. Anticholinester-ase then has no effect on the patient, and the muscle fatigue persists.

A cholinergic crisis occurs when there is too high a level of anticholin-esterase in the system. It may cause respiratory paralysis. The condition is reversible with atropine. To identify a cholinergic crisis, *REMEMBER:*

- Red as a beet (vasodilation)
- Mad as a hatter (neurologic changes)
- Hotter than hell (core temperature rises)
- Dry as a bone (saliva decreases, no sweating)

(continued)

Normal:

Nerve impulse → ACh liberated → depolarization → muscle contracts
       ↓
     (a neurotransmitter)

Abnormal:

Nerve impulse → ACH liberated *but*
         ↓
       → Cholinesterase destroys ACh → muscle weakness

 Rx: Anticholinesterase (neostigmine, Mestinon) to destroy antibodies.

Figure 1-23 Myasthenia gravis diagram.

● NERVE STIMULATOR

When administering neuromuscular blocking agents, a peripheral nerve stimulator is used to monitor the level of blockade. Electrical stimulation is applied to either the ulnar nerve, facial nerve, or posterior tibial nerve, with the ulnar nerve being the preferred site.

1. Place electrodes along ulnar nerve, 3 to 5 cm apart.

2. Apply alligator clips to electrodes (polarity is insignificant).

3. Press TOF (train of four) to elicit four mild electrical stimuli.

4. Goal is usually to have patient respond with one twitch out of four stimuli.

 a. Zero twitches = decrease neuromuscular blockade

 b. Two twitches = increase neuromuscular blockade

Note: Determine amount of current required to produce four strong responses as a baseline before starting neuromuscular blocking agent, and increase by 10% when using drug therapy.

(continued)

NOTES

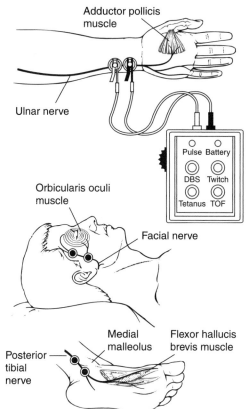

Pulse Battery

DBS Twitch

Tetanus TOF

FIGURE 1-24 Nerve stimulator. (Courtesy of Neuro Technology, Inc., Houston, TX).

○ NEUROGENIC HYPERVENTILATION (see Central Neurogenic Hyperventilation and Respiratory Patterns in Part 3, Pulmonary System)

○ NEURONS

Neurons are composed of a cell body and two types of processes: axons and dendrites. An axon is a single extension carrying impulses **away** from the cell body. Dendrites (meaning "tree like") are processes carrying impulses **toward** the cell body. There is only **one** axon, but several dendrites. A myelin sheath (made by Schwann cells) surrounds some axons. The nodes of Ranvier are areas along the axon not covered by myelin. They increase the speed of conduction. Synaptic knobs are the end portions where acetylcholine and epinephrine are stored.

(continued)

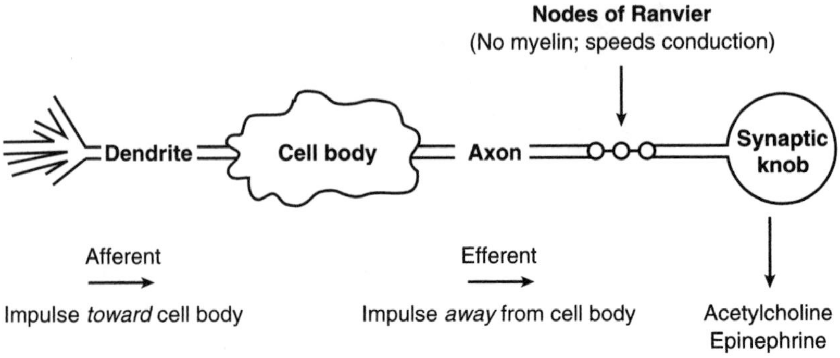

Nodes of Ranvier
(No myelin; speeds conduction)

Dendrite — Cell body — Axon —O-O-O— Synaptic knob

Afferent → Impulse *toward* cell body

Efferent → Impulse *away* from cell body

Acetylcholine
Epinephrine

FIGURE **1-25** A neuron.

The **upper motor neurons** conduct impulses from the brain to the spinal cord (or head to spine). The **lower motor neurons** conduct impulses from muscles to the spinal cord (or periphery to spine). The upper motor neurons (brain to spinal cord) do not have to be involved when attempting to elicit a reflex. Therefore, an exaggerated reflex indicates a problem. However, lower motor neurons (periphery to cord) are essential to the reflex, and if no response is elicited, it indicates a lower motor neuron problem.

REMEMBER:

Upper neurons (superior) = spastic
Lower neurons (floor level) = flaccid

NEUROTRANSMITTERS (see also Myasthenia Gravis)

Acetylcholine is the major transmitter at the neuromuscular junction. Other neurotransmitters are (1) norepinephrine, (2) dopamine, and (3) serotonin.

NUCHAL RIGIDITY (see also Brudzinski's Sign)

Nuchal rigidity occurs in meningeal irritation and produces pain and stiffness when attempting to flex the head to the chest.

OCULOCEPHALIC REFLEX (see Doll's Eyes)

⬤ OCULOVESTIBULAR REFLEX (see Caloric Test)

⬤ OLIGODENDROGLIOMA (see Tumors, Neurogenic)

⬤ OPISTHOTONOS

Extension of the body with the neck and back arched is opisthotonos. It is seen in patients with tetany or with damage to brain stem.

⬤ PARKINSON'S DISEASE (see also Stereotactic Surgery)

Rigidity, masklike face, shuffling gait, and tremors of Parkinson's disease are related to deficiency of dopamine in basal ganglia. Dopamine itself does not cross the blood-brain barrier; therefore, L-dopa, a precursor of dopamine, must be given as a replacement. Stereotactic surgery is sometimes helpful.

⬤ PINEAL REGION TUMORS (see Tumors, Neurogenic)

⬤ PITUITARY ADENOMA (See Tumors, Neurogenic)

⬤ PLASMAPHERESIS

Plasmapheresis is removal of one or more components of blood after the blood is separated into component parts. Access is established via a large-bore, double-lumen central venous line or a large antecubital vein, and the patient is connected to an extracorporeal circuit. The "old" plasma is removed from whole blood by flow through a cell separator, where it is centrifuged down (or passed through a microporous membrane filter) and exchanged for "new" plasma in the form of replacement fluid. (There is an alternate method whereby the plasma is separated out, filtered to remove the disease mediator, then returned to the patient.) In both methods, because the extracorporeal circuit contains 150 to 400 mL of blood during the procedure, the patient needs to be able to tolerate the low volume. It is used in myasthenia gravis or Guillain-Barré syndrome to remove autoantibodies, as well as in other immune-related disorders such as multiple myeloma, lupus, or rheumatoid arthritis.

⬤ PONS

The pons consists of fibers and nuclei situated at the base of the brain that receive impulses from the cerebral cortex. A lesion in the pons is accompanied by pinpoint pupils and apneustic breathing.

⬤ **POSTURING (see Decerebrate, Decorticate, Opisthotonos)**

⬤ **PUPIL GAUGE**

1 mm   2 mm   3 mm   4 mm   5 mm

6 mm   7 mm   8 mm   9 mm   10 mm   FIGURE 1-26 Pupil gauge.

⬤ **RACCOON EYES (see Basilar Skull Fracture)**

⬤ **RETICULAR ACTIVATING SYSTEM**

Reticular activating system is essential for arousal from sleep, alert wakefulness, focusing of attention, and perceptual association. Destructive lesions of upper pons and midbrain produce coma.

⬤ **RINNE TEST (see also Caloric Test, Weber's Test)**

The Rinne test is used to diagnose middle ear disease by testing the eighth cranial nerve. Place vibrating tuning fork on mastoid bone. When sound is no longer heard, fork is placed in front of the ear, where sound is normally louder (conduction through bone versus through air).

⬤ **ROMBERG'S TEST**

This tests for cerebellar dysfunction. Patient is asked to stand with legs together, arms out, eyes closed. Any swaying movement indicates a problem, because the cerebellum is responsible for coordination.

⬤ **SCHWANNOMA (see Tumors, Neurogenic)**

··

◖ SEIZURES

A seizure is an electrical discharge in the neurons of the cerebral cortex and possibly neurons of the brain stem. The etiology or precipitating factors are many, including genes, cerebral tumors, metabolic disorders, AV malformations of the brain, trauma, infections, and cerebral vascular disease, to name a few.

Treatment involves first preventing injury during seizure activity and protecting the airway. Improved control of seizure activity by monitoring and maintaining therapeutic drug levels must follow. (See also Therapeutic Drug Levels in Part 10, Labs.)

TABLE 1-6. Common Seizure Drugs

· ·

Drug	Used for	Therapeutic Level
Phenytoin (Dilantin)	Generalized or partial	10–20 μg/ml
Phenobarbital	Generalized or partial	15–40 μg/ml
Primidone (Mysoline)	Generalized and complex	7–15 μg/ml
Carbamazepine (Tegretol)	Generalized and simple or complex	8–12 μg/ml
Clonazepam (Klonopin)	Myoclonic and akinetic	40–100 μg/ml
Ethosuximide (Zarontin)	Petit mal and complex partial	40–90 μg/ml

PARTIAL SEIZURE	Initial neuronal discharge is limited to **one** focal site or **one** cerebral hemisphere. Clinical symptoms usually begin on one side of body. Partial seizures may progress into generalized seizures.
• Simple partial	No impaired level of consciousness.
• Complex partial	Impaired level of consciousness. Inability to respond to external stimuli. No memory of event. Repeat of inappropriate acts called automatisms, such as smacking of lips, chewing movements.
GENERALIZED SEIZURE	The manifestations of this type of seizure are seen bilaterally and in both hemispheres.
• Absence (petit mal)	Sudden loss of awareness. Mostly in children, sometimes as many as 300 in 24 hours.
• Generalized motor (grand mal)	Tonic movement (abrupt increase in muscle tone) and clonic movement (jerky, rhythmic movement) to both sides of body.
• Status epilepticus	Persistent seizure activity lasting 30 minutes or longer. Sometimes alternates with periods of unconsciousness.
• Myoclonic	Sudden, brief muscular contractions that may occur singly or repetitively; usually involves arms.
• Akinetic	Sudden, brief loss of muscle tone; "drop attacks."

⬤ **SKULL FRACTURE** (see Basilar Skull Fracture)

⬤ **SPINAL CORD** (see also Lumbar Puncture, Spinal Injury, Vertebrae)

The spinal cord extends from the foramen magnum to the second lumbar vertebra. The anterior gray column (anterior horn) contains efferent or motor fibers. The posterior gray column (posterior horn) contains cell bodies of the afferent or sensory fibers. The lateral column (prominent in upper cervical, thoracic, and midsacral regions) contains preganglionic fibers of the autonomic nervous system. The white matter, arranged into three longitudinal columns called anterior, lateral, and posterior funiculi, contain mostly myelinated axons. The funiculi also contain tracts that are functionally distinct (ie, have the same or similar origin, course, and termination) and are classified as ascending or descending.

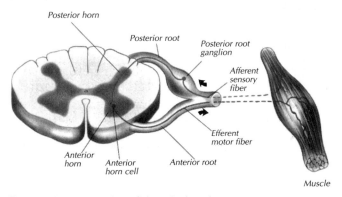

FIGURE 1-27 Cross section of the spinal cord.

The major *ascending* tracts of the spinal cord (afferent, sensory, posterior) (see Fig. 1-28) are pathways *to the brain* for impulses entering the cord via the dorsal root of the spinal nerves.

1. Fasciculus gracilis and fasciculus cuneatus convey sensations of position, movement, touch, and pressure.

2. Lateral spinothalamic tract conveys sensations of pain and temperature.

3. Ventral spinothalamic tract transmits stimuli of touch and pressure.

4. Dorsal spinocerebellar tract conveys sensory impulses from muscles and muscle tendons to cerebellum.

5. Ventral spinocerebellar tract is same as dorsal spinocerebellar tract.

6. Spinotectal tract pathway correlates with pathway of spinal cord.

(continued)

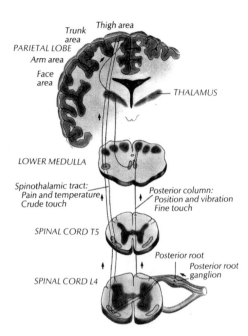

Trunk area
Thigh area
PARIETAL LOBE
Arm area
Face area
THALAMUS
LOWER MEDULLA
Spinothalamic tract:
Pain and temperature
Crude touch
Posterior column:
Position and vibration
Fine touch
SPINAL CORD T5
Posterior root
Posterior root ganglion
SPINAL CORD L4

FIGURE 1-28 Major *ascending* tracts of the spinal cord.

The major *descending* tracts of the spinal cord (efferent, motor, anterior) (see Fig. 1-29) transmit impulses *from the brain* to the motor neurons of the spinal cord.

1. Corticospinal (pyramidal) tract is the major pathway from the cortex to the peripheral motor nerves for voluntary movement.

2. Tectospinal tract mediates optic and auditory reflexes.

3. Rubrospinal tract conveys impulses from the cerebellum to the anterior column motor cells.

(*continued*)

NOTES

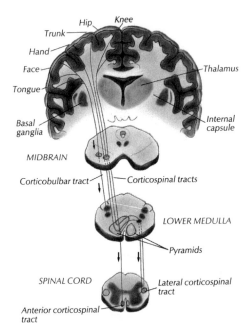

FIGURE 1-29 Major *descending* tracts of the spinal cord.

⬤ **SPINAL INJURY (see also Brown-Séquard's Syndrome, Lumbar Puncture, Spinal Cord, Vertebrae)**

The degree and location of injury to the spinal cord determine the extent of the disability. If the injury is high in the cervical region, respiratory failure and death follow paralysis of the diaphragm. *(REMEMBER:* **C3, 4, 5 keep the diaphragm alive.)** Midcervical injuries result in breathing only by diaphragmatic movement, because the muscles of the upper thorax are paralyzed. Thoracic vertebrae are seldom injured because they are protected by the rib cage. The fifth and sixth cervical vertebrae and the first and fifth lumbar vertebrae are especially vulnerable, and injury to the cord at these levels is frequent. The severity of injury to the cord also determines how much function is lost. When the cord is completely severed, function is lost permanently below the level of the injury. If the damage to the cord is partial, some function may be maintained or, at times, even regained.

(continued)

TABLE 1-7. Location of Spinal Cord Injury and Related Disability

Injury to	Findings
C1, C2, C3	Usually fatal.
C4	Quadraplegia, respiration difficulty.
C5–C8	Variable function of neck, shoulder, and arm muscles.
T1–T11	Paraplegia. Respiration is a concern because upper thoracic region innervates intercostal muscles. Loss of vasomotor tone, vagal responses. Inability to regulate heart rate. Loss of autonomic nerve impulses. Occasionally, leg braces can be used when injury is to lower thoracic spine.
T12–L3	Paraplegia. Mixed picture of motor and sensory loss, bowel and bladder dysfunction. Probable wheelchair; leg braces necessary.

◖ SPINAL SHOCK

The first picture of a patient with spinal cord injury is one of spinal shock. The cord is "jolted" so that nothing works, and the patient is areflexic with flaccid paralysis below the level of the injury, including loss of pain and sensation below the level of the injury, anhydrous below the level of the injury, and bowel and bladder dysfunction below the level of the injury. The duration can be days, weeks, or months. Interventions include close monitoring of the respiratory status. Blood pressure may drop, and if it does, there is probably damage to the thoracic area or above. Bradycardia (vagus nerve) as well as decreased temperature and decreased potassium levels may also be seen.

◖ STATUS EPILEPTICUS (see Seizures)

◖ STEREOGNOSIS

Stereognosis is tactile discrimination, or recognizing the form and size of objects by touch. It is determined by parietal lobe function.

◖ STEREOTACTIC SURGERY

Stereotactic surgery (*stereo* = three dimensional; *tactic* = to touch) is based on atlases of three-dimensional coordinates compiled from dissections. Current techniques would be more appropriately termed image-guided stereotactic surgery, as a CT scan, an MRI, or occasionally an angiogram is performed with a compatible device affixed to the patient's head, allowing the target to be precisely localized.

(continued)

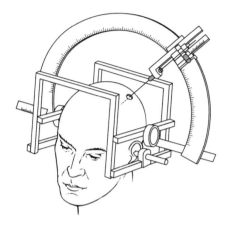

FIGURE 1-30 Stereotactic frame. (Reprinted with permission. CIBA Collection of Medical Illustrations [1991]. *Neurology and neurosurgery* [Vol I, Part II.]. New York: Churchill Livingstone.)

Many different frames have been developed, the most common of which are the Leksell, Todd-Wells, Brown-Robert-Wells, and Guiot. Then a set of guides, oriented to the same coordinate system, are used to direct biopsy needles and so forth to the target location. This method is useful for biopsy or aspiration of small, deeply situated tumors or abscesses. When stereotactics are combined with craniotomy, it provides for a more direct localization and obviates the need for ventriculography.

Brown-Robert-Wells (BRW) system:

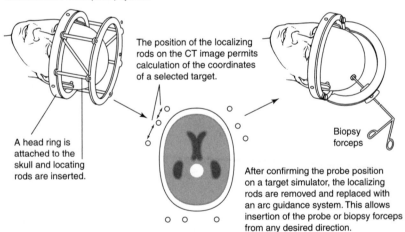

The position of the localizing rods on the CT image permits calculation of the coordinates of a selected target.

A head ring is attached to the skull and locating rods are inserted.

Biopsy forceps

After confirming the probe position on a target simulator, the localizing rods are removed and replaced with an arc guidance system. This allows insertion of the probe or biopsy forceps from any desired direction.

FIGURE 1-31 Stereotactic procedure. (Reprinted with permission. Lindsey, K., Bone, I., & Callender, R. [1991]. *Neurology and neurosurgery illustrated* [2nd ed.]. New York: Churchill Livingstone.)

◯ SUBARACHNOID BOLT (see Intracranial Pressure Monitoring)

◯ SUBARACHNOID HEMORRHAGE (see also Aneurysms, Arteriovenous Malformation, Transcranial Doppler Studies, Vasospasm)

Subarachnoid hemorrhage (SAH) is caused by the rupture of an aneurysm, trauma, tumor, or arteriovenous malformation. The patient presents with a classic triad of symptoms: (1) sudden explosive headache, (2) decreased level of consciousness, and (3) nuchal rigidity. In addition, SAH is well known to cause EKG changes in the ST segment and the T wave, with a prominent U wave.

- **Vasospasm risk:** 40% to 60% incidence with 20% to 30% of patient's showing symptoms. Can begin anytime, most likely 5 to 7 days *postbleed* (not postop). Usually resolves by day 21. Diagnosed by transcranial Doppler studies and/or arteriogram.
- **Rebleed risk:** A rebleed is possible 7 to 10 days after the initial bleed, with peak incidence on days 4 through 8. This is the greatest cause of death.

◯ SUBDURAL HEMATOMA

Subdural hematoma is usually caused by a *venous* bleed causing blood to accumulate between the dura mater and arachnoid layers. It is often related to trauma. Patient will appear sleepy with a decreased level of consciousness, similar to a TIA. The pupil on the side of the lesion is usually dilated. The onset of the symptoms is slow: for an acute bleed, 24 to 72 hours is common; for a subacute bleed, 48 to 72 hours. A chronic, slow bleed can take up to several weeks postinjury to manifest symptoms. Diagnosis is confirmed by CT scan.

◯ TENTORIUM CEREBELLI

A tentorium is a fold made by dura mater, between the occipital lobe and cerebellum. It is used as a line of demarcation.

◯ TRANSCRANIAL DOPPLER STUDIES

Utilizing an ultrasound beam directed into a column of blood, transcranial Doppler studies measure the velocity of red blood cells at a specific depth and at specific sites. It is a noninvasive test, quick to administer, and easily repeatable.

(*continued*)

Normal velocities	MCA 50–60 cm/sec
	AC 30–40 cm/sec
Criteria	120 cm/sec, bears watching
	140–170 cm/sec, mild to moderate vasospasm
	170–250 cm/sec, moderate to severe vasospasm
	>250 cm/sec, trouble (angioplasty?)

TROUSSEAU'S SIGN (see also Chvostek's Sign)

Apply sphygmomanometer cuff to upper arm and inflate until radial pulse is obliterated. Keep inflated for about 3 minutes. A positive sign is evidenced by spasm of the lower arm and hand muscles (carpal spasm), indicating hypocalcemia. If there is no spasm, the sign is negative.

TUMORS, NEUROGENIC

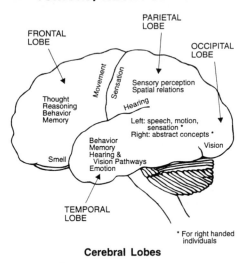

Figure 1-32 Cerebral function and associated anatomical areas. (Reproduced with permission from the American Brain Tumor Association.)

- **Acoustic neuroma (Schwannoma):** A benign tumor of the eighth cranial nerve (hearing) located in the posterior fossa. It commonly occurs in adults, usually in their middle years. Symptoms are loss of hearing of one ear, buzzing or ringing in the ear (tinnitus), and occasionally some dizziness. If the tumor also affects the adjacent seventh cranial nerve (facial nerve), some facial paralysis, difficulty in swallowing, loss of sensation in the face, impaired eye movement, and unsteadiness may occur. In most cases, this tumor can be completely removed by surgery. After surgery, there may be per-
  (continued)

manent or temporary damage to the facial nerve resulting in some facial paralysis.

- **Adenoma:** (see Pituitary Adenoma, below)
- **Astrocytoma:** A tumor of the supportive (glial) tissue of the brain. It may be benign or malignant, graded I through III. Grade III tumors are called anaplastic astrocytomas. Grade IV tumors are designated glioblastomas. The benign astrocytoma (Grade I or II) is a slow-growing tumor, but it may infiltrate some large areas. Sometimes, this tumor may be encapsulated in a cyst. The usual treatment for malignant forms of this tumor is partial or complete removal by surgery, followed by radiation therapy.
- **Craniopharyngioma:** A benign, congenital tumor, cystic in nature, commonly occurring in children. The tumor usually appears in the midline suprasellar region, involving the third ventricle, optic nerve, and pituitary gland. Surgery is the common treatment for this type of tumor, and it may be completely removed if it is in a favorable location. Radiation therapy may be administered if the tumor is not completely removed.
- **Ependymoma:** A childhood tumor appearing in the posterior fossa and in the cerebral hemisphere. It may be benign or malignant and is usually slow growing. Occasionally, these tumors may seed to other locations in the nervous system. They usually are not totally removable by surgery because of their position in the brain (floor of the fourth ventricle or deep in the cerebral hemisphere). Treatment consists of radiation and a shunt to relieve the increased ICP. Often, chemotherapy is used.
- **Glioblastoma:** A Grade IV tumor rarely controlled by surgery because the cells of the tumor frequently stray throughout the brain. Thus, radiation therapy is almost always used following surgery or biopsy, followed by aggressive chemotherapy. Although many tumors contain a mixture of cells, this one is especially hard to treat because while one cell type may be responsive to treatment and die off, other types are waiting in the wings to take over.
- **Glioma:** (see Astrocytoma, Oligodendroglioma, Glioblastoma) A general "family" name for a variety of different types of tumor of the glial (supportive) tissue of the brain.
- **Medulloblastoma:** A rapidly growing, malignant tumor of the cerebellum, occurring mainly in children. It is an invasive tumor, frequently metastatic via the spinal fluid. Surgical removal followed by radiation of the tumor area and the entire brain and spinal cord is the treatment of choice. The tumor is very radiosensitive and is

(continued)

often cured by this treatment alone. Recurrent tumors may be treated with chemotherapy.

- **Oligodendroglioma:** As with astrocytomas, these are tumors of the supportive (glial) tissue of the brain. They most frequently occur in middle-aged individuals and are usually located in the cerebral hemispheres. They are generally slow growing and benign, although malignant forms are possible. Often they are present for many years before diagnosis and permit survival for years afterward. Treatment consists of surgical removal of as much of the tumor as possible, followed by a course of radiation. Recurrence is not unusual.

- **Pineal region tumors:** Usual treatment for these tumors is radiation due to the fact that the surgical approach is very difficult. The tumors are generally very responsive to the radiation, and a shunt procedure is also generally done to relieve increased intracranial pressure. Often this treatment is curative.

- **Pituitary adenoma:** Tumors of the pituitary gland commonly occur in young or middle-aged adults. Treatment typically consists of surgical removal and is often curative. Other treatment may include various forms of radiation or drug therapy.

UNCAL HERNIATION (see Herniation)

VASOSPASM

Vasospasm is a sustained constriction or narrowing of a cerebral artery or arteries subsequent to a subarachnoid bleed. The spasms cause ischemia and decreased cerebral blood flow, and they play a major part in determining the patient's overall outcome. They occur in 40% to 60% of all patients with SAH, with 20% to 30% showing symptoms, which vary from mild to severe. Diagnosis is by transcranial Doppler studies or angiogram. It has been shown that an internal carotid aneurysm has a greater propensity to produce vasospasm than an MCA. Also of note is that a decreased sodium level increases the chance of spasm, because less sodium creates less fluid as it takes H_2O with it. Research to date has failed to provide evidence as to the reason for the spasms, and it remains unclear if the vasospasm is a normal or abnormal contraction, if it is a failure of arterial smooth muscle cells to relax, or whether it represents a thickening in the vessel wall.

- **Peak incidence:** Day 5 to 7 *postbleed* (not postsurgery), but can occur from day 1 to 21.

(*continued*)

▪ **Treatment:**

Angioplasty	An attempt to improve blood flow by dilating vessels interfering with circulation via a balloon-tip.
Calcium channel blockers	Nimotop (nimodipine) has been shown to have a special affinity for cerebral vessels. Although it does not appear to affect the severity of spasms, it has demonstrated an improved patient outcome overall.
Hemodilution	Allows easier blood flow past site of constriction. Give fluids to reduce hematocrit to approximately 30%.
Hypervolemia	Crystalloids, colloids (albumin, Plasmanate). Keep CVP up to 10 mmHg; PCWP 16 to 18.
Hypertension	Dopamine, dobutamine, and/or Levophed. Keep SBP 160 to 220.
Papaverine	A smooth muscle relaxant; possibly works by blocking calcium channels. Injected during angioplasty.

VENTRICULOSTOMY (see Intracranial Pressure Monitoring)

VERTEBRAE (see also Lumbar Puncture, Spinal Cord, Spinal Injury)

Referred to as 26 in number (not 33), vertebrae are named and numbered from above downward:

(*continued*)

NOTES

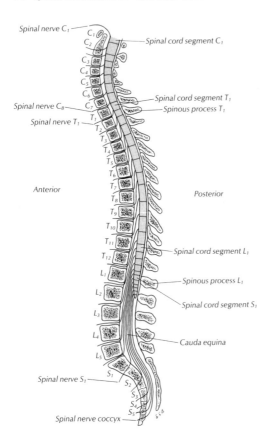

Spinal nerve C_1

Spinal cord segment C_1

Spinal nerve C_8

Spinal cord segment T_1

Spinous process T_1

Spinal nerve T_1

Anterior

Posterior

Spinal cord segment L_1

Spinous process L_1

Spinal cord segment S_1

Cauda equina

Spinal nerve S_1

Spinal nerve coccyx

FIGURE 1-33 The vertebrae.

7 cervical

12 thoracic

5 lumbar

1 sacral (5 sacral fused by adulthood to form 1)

1 coccygeal (4 coccygeal united firmly to form 1)

WEBER'S TEST (see also Caloric Test, Rinne Test)

This is an acoustic test for eighth cranial nerve. Vibrating tuning fork is placed on middle of patient's forehead. Hearing sound equally in both ears is a normal finding. If sound balance is skewed, impaired function of the cochlear nerve is suspected.

Cardiovascular System

🔘 ACTION POTENTIAL

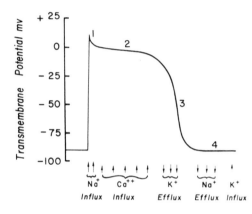

Figure 2-1 Action potential of human ventricular myocardium together with probable electrolyte movements. (Schlant, R.C., & Alexander, R.W. [1994]. *Hurst's the heart* [8th ed.]. New York: McGraw-Hill. Reprinted with permission of the McGraw-Hill Companies.)

Phase 0: Rapid Depolarization (sodium in)

On depolarization, the cell becomes permeable to sodium through "fast" channels, and sodium, previously outside the cell, rushes inside. This causes the initial rapid upstroke of the curve and a reversal of potential (resting cell was negative on the inside and becomes positive on the inside when depolarized).

Phase 1: Initial Repolarization (sodium stops, chloride in)

The brief, rapid start of repolarization is believed to be due to the inactivation of the inbound sodium as well as a secondary influx of chloride.

Phase 2: Repolarization Plateau (calcium in, potassium out)

The repolarization slows as a result of a complex interaction between a slow influx of calcium entering the cell and a slow exiting of potassium. Phases 1 and 2 are periods of absolute refractoriness.

Phase 3: Repolarization Continues (calcium stops, potassium out)

The influx of calcium ceases, while the outward flow of potassium continues. Phase 3 is a period of relative refractoriness.

(continued)

Phase 4: Resting (sodium/potassium pump)

Most cardiac cells are −70 to −90 mV at rest. The net negative electrical charge is restored by a sodium/potassium exchange across the membrane. The slow diastolic depolarization is caused by a time-dependent fall in outbound potassium. This, combined with an increase in the sodium influx, causes the threshold to be reached.

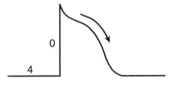

FIGURE 2-2 Action potential memory aid. Remember, once you hit 40, it's downhill!

ALLEN'S TEST

Elevate patient's hand with fist clenched while both radial and ulnar arteries are compressed to occlude arterial blood flow. Pressure is then released over only the ulnar artery. Color should return to the hand within 6 seconds, indicating a patent ulnar artery and adequate collateral blood flow to the hand.

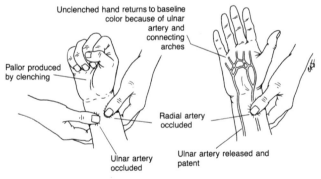

FIGURE 2-3 Allen's test.

ARTERIAL PRESSURE (see Intraarterial Pressure)

NOTES

⬤ ASHMAN'S PHENOMENON

Ashman's theory states that aberrant conduction is more likely to complicate atrial fibrillation when a longer cycle is succeeded by a shorter one:

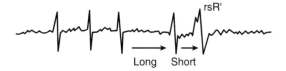

rsR'

Long   Short

FIGURE 2-4 Ashman's phenomenon: atrial fibrillation with long-short-long cycle.

The phenomenon may also occur when sinus bradycardia is complicated by a PAC. Cycle of sinus bradycardia is long, but PAC shortens cycle and is conducted aberrantly (usually in RBB pattern, rsR'):

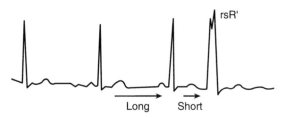

rsR'

Long   Short

FIGURE 2-5 Ashman's phenomenon: sinus bradycardia with PAC.

Therefore, according to Ashman, *the beat that follows a long/short cycle favors aberrancy.* This, however, is not a hard, fast rule, because by the rule of bigeminy, a longer cycle also tends to produce a ventricular ectopic beat equally as many times.

⬤ AXIS DEVIATION

The axis is the mean direction (vector) in which electrical activity spreads across the heart. The strength of the vector is indicated by recording a small deflection for a weak vector and a large deflection for a strong vector.

Normal axis is described by some authors to be in the narrow bounds of $+30°$ to $+60°$ and by others to be between $0°$ and $+90°$. Using the range from $-30°$ to $+110°$ allows easier definition of hemiblock.

(continued)

NOTES

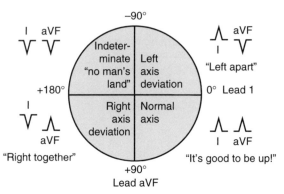

FIGURE 2-6 Determining electrical axis. (Adapted from Hudak, C.M., Gallo, B.M., & Morton, P.G. [1998]. *Critical care nursing* [7th ed.]. Philadelphia: Lippincott-Raven.)

Quick Method for Determining Axis

1. Examine deflections in leads I and aVF.

2. If they point toward each other on the 12-lead EKG (lead I negative, aVF positive), the deviation is to the right.

3. If they point away from each other on the 12-lead EKG (lead I positive, aVF negative), the deviation is to the left.

REMEMBER: **The axis is "right together" or "left apart."**

4. If both leads I and aVF deviate upward, the axis is normal.

REMEMBER: **It's good to be up!**

5. If both leads I and aVF deviate downward, the axis is in "no man's land" or indeterminate (usually due to a junctional rhythm).

(continued)

NOTES

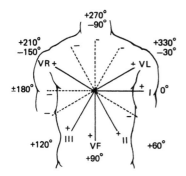

FIGURE 2-7 Hexiaxial figure to pinpoint axis. (Goldman, M.J. [1996]. *Principles of clinical electrocardiography* [12th ed.]. Los Altos, CA: Lange Medical Publications. Reprinted with permission.)

More Exact, Hexaxial Method for Determining Axis

1. Find the most equiphasic lead (lead that equals zero when the value of the positive and negative deflections are added) using leads I, II, III, aVR, aVL, and aVF. (No V leads!)

2. Use the hexaxial figure to determine which lead is perpendicular to the equiphasic one.

3. Check if the QRS of this lead is a negative or positive deflection. This gives the direction of the vector.

If there is no equiphasic deflection present in the six limb leads:

• Look at leads I and aVF to place the axis in one of the quadrants.

• Determine which of the other two leads in that quadrant have the largest complex and place the axis closest to that vector.

Hints:

• V tach commonly has an axis in no man's land, giving a clue to the differential diagnosis between ventricular ectopy and aberration.

• Axis shifts to the left with age. An axis of −30° is not necessarily a cardiac disorder.

• ALL complexes in the V lead deflecting either up or down are definitive of V tach.

• Axis deviates **toward** bundle branch block (RBBB = R axis deviation).

• Axis deviates **away** from MI.

Left Axis Deviation Caused by	Right Axis Deviation Caused by
• Advanced age, obesity, pregnancy	• Youth, tall and thin body form
• Left ventricular hypertrophy	• Right ventricular hypertrophy
• Inferior MI	• COPD, pulmonary emboli, infarcts
• WPW syndrome	• Dextrocardia
• Ascites, tumors	

⬤ BODY SURFACE AREA NOMOGRAM

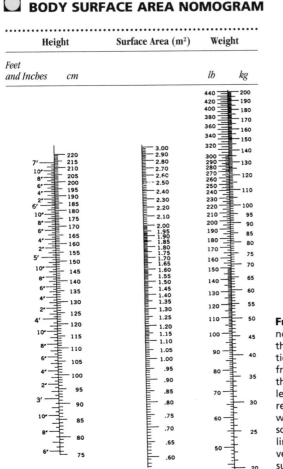

Height	Surface Area (m²)	Weight

FIGURE 2-8 Body surface area nomogram. To determine the surface area of the patient, draw a straight line from the point representing the patient's height on the left vertical scale to the point representing the patient's weight on the right vertical scale. The point at which this line intersects the middle vertical scale represents the surface area in square meters.

⬤ CABG (see Cardiac Surgery, Postop Considerations)

NOTES

CARDIAC ENZYMES

Enzyme	Onset	Peak	Return to Normal
CK	3–6 hr	12–24 hr	3–5 days
CK-MB	2–4 hr	12–20 hr	48–72 hr
LDH	24 hr	48–72 hr	7–10 days
LDH$_1$	4 hr	48 hr	10 days
LDH$_2$	4 hr	48 hr	10 days

Troponin I
  Healthy individuals have undetectable troponin. Typical AMI patients commonly have values greater than 10 ng/mL. Lesser ischemic insults extend to the lower level of detectability (0.4 ng/mL) in a continuous spectrum. Follow serially, comparable to CKMB. Troponin elevation can usually be detected within 4 hours after an acute MI and can remain elevated for 1–2 weeks.

FIGURE 2-9 Cardiac enzyme patterns. (Adapted from Smeltzer, S.C., & Bare, B.G. [1996]. *Brunner and Suddarth's textbook of medical-surgical nursing* [8th ed.]. Philadelphia: Lippincott-Raven.)

CARDIAC INDEX (see Swan-Ganz: Hemodynamic Normals)

N O T E S

CARDIAC SURGERY, POSTOP CONSIDERATIONS

Proposed algorithm for adult patients:

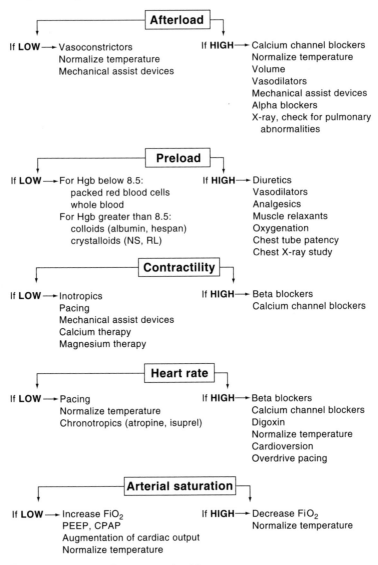

Afterload

If **LOW** → Vasoconstrictors
Normalize temperature
Mechanical assist devices

If **HIGH** → Calcium channel blockers
Normalize temperature
Volume
Vasodilators
Mechanical assist devices
Alpha blockers
X-ray, check for pulmonary
abnormalities

Preload

If **LOW** → For Hgb below 8.5:
packed red blood cells
whole blood
For Hgb greater than 8.5:
colloids (albumin, hespan)
crystalloids (NS, RL)

If **HIGH** → Diuretics
Vasodilators
Analgesics
Muscle relaxants
Oxygenation
Chest tube patency
Chest X-ray study

Contractility

If **LOW** → Inotropics
Pacing
Mechanical assist devices
Calcium therapy
Magnesium therapy

If **HIGH** → Beta blockers
Calcium channel blockers

Heart rate

If **LOW** → Pacing
Normalize temperature
Chronotropics (atropine, isuprel)

If **HIGH** → Beta blockers
Calcium channel blockers
Digoxin
Normalize temperature
Cardioversion
Overdrive pacing

Arterial saturation

If **LOW** → Increase FiO_2
PEEP, CPAP
Augmentation of cardiac output
Normalize temperature

If **HIGH** → Decrease FiO_2
Normalize temperature

FIGURE 2-10 Post–cardiac surgery algorithm.

General principles for weaning drips: Policies vary widely from institution to institution. These are general guidelines only.

- **Dobutrex:** Keep initially, wean later
  Dobutrex is not used for BP, but in low cardiac output states. It increases contractility, CO and decreases wedge pressure, SVR.

- **Nitroglycerine:** Keep initially, wean later
  Nitroglycerine is used for the "ischemic heart." High dose of 50 to 250 μg/kg increases cardiac output and decreases SVR, wedge pressure, and CVP. Low dose of 20 to 40 μg/kg causes no change in CO or SVR but decreases wedge pressure and CVP.

- **Dopamine:** Wean as appropriate
  Dopamine increases contractility, cardiac output, SVR, and CVP, but it also increases O_2 consumption.

- **Nipride:** Wean as appropriate
  Nipride is used for hypertension secondary to ischemic heart. It decreases CVP, SVR.

- **Epinephrine:** Wean as appropriate
  Epinephrine strengthens myocardial contraction, increases BP, and increases cardiac output. It also accelerates heart rate.

◻ **CARDIAC TAMPONADE** (see Tamponade)

◻ **CARDIOGENIC SHOCK** (see Shock, Cardiogenic)

NOTES

◐ COARCTATION OF THE AORTA

Aortic constriction, usually distal to the left subclavian artery, stresses the left ventricle and causes an increase in afterload. A graft is often required to repair it.

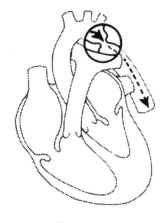

FIGURE 2-11 Coarctation of the aorta.

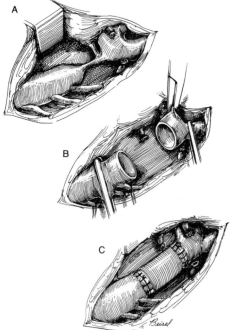

FIGURE 2-12 Surgical repair of coarctation of the aorta using a tubular graft prosthesis. **(A)** The coarctation is exposed through a left lateral thoracotomy incision. **(B)** Clamps are applied to the aorta above and below the area of coarctation and the coarcted segment is excised. **(C)** A tubular prosthetic graft is placed to bridge the defect and sutured to the aorta in end-to-end fashion. (Waldhausen, J.A., Pierce, W.S., & Campbell, D.B. [Eds.]. [1996] *Surgery of the chest* [6th ed]. St. Louis: Mosby, Inc. Reprinted with permission.)

⬤ COR PULMONALE

Right-sided heart failure with the following hallmarks:

- Tall peak P waves in leads II, III, and aVF
- T wave inversion
- ST segment changes
- Right axis deviation
- Right ventricular hypertrophy
- Low voltage on EKG
- Conduction defects

⬤ CORONARY ARTERIES

Right coronary artery perfuses:	Left anterior descending (LAD) artery perfuses:
SA node in 60% of population AV node in 80–90% of population Bundle of HIS Part of left bundle branch Posterior third of septum Right atrium and ventricle Inferior wall of left ventricle	Anterior wall of left ventricle Two-thirds of septum Right bundle branch Part of left bundle branch
	Left circumflex (LCA) artery perfuses:
	Part of the left bundle branch Lateral wall of left atrium and ventricle SA node of 40% of population

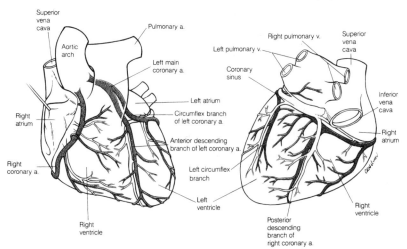

FIGURE 2-13 Coronary circulation: coronary arteries and some coronary sinus veins.

○ **CVP (see Swan-Ganz: Hemodynamic Normals)**

○ **DEFIBRILLATION**

Energy stored in the defibrillator is constant, so the only variance to the delivered current is due to the operator and the impedance of the individual patient's chest. To minimize this variance:

• Cover electrodes with the appropriate paste or gel, or use pads to provide the lowest resistance.

• Use 25 pounds of pressure per paddle.

• Use proper paddle placement so that the heart (primarily the ventricles) is in the path of the current.

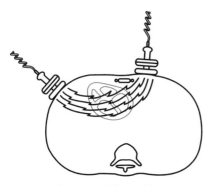 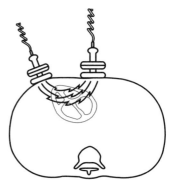

Correct paddle position	Incorrect paddle position
(current passes through the ventricles)	(current misses part of the ventricles)

FIGURE 2-14 Correct and incorrect paddle placement for defibrillation. (Crockett, P. *Defib: What you should know.* [1991]. Redmond, WA: Physio-Control. Reprinted with permission.)

(continued)

NOTES

The sternum/apex position is most frequently used, with the sternum paddle on the upper right chest to the right of the sternum, below the clavicle, and the apex paddle on the lower left chest over the cardiac apex, to the left of the nipple in the midaxillary line.

To defibrillate a patient with an implanted pacemaker:

Place the paddles as far away from the pulse generator as possible. Standard anterior/lateral placement is most convenient, but it delivers defibrillation energy in the same direction as the pacemaker's sensing vector and may damage the pacemaker. Place the paddles in the anterior/ posterior position so energy is delivered perpendicular to the sensing vector.

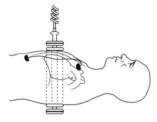

FIGURE 2-15 Anterior/posterior paddle placement for patients with an implanted pacemaker. (Crockett, P. *Defib: What you should know.* [1991]. Redmond, WA: Physio-Control. Reprinted with permission.)

To defibrillate a patient with an implanted defibrillator:

If an unconscious patient receives shocks from an implanted defibrillator but V-tach or V-fib persist, external countershock should be delivered. It is possible that the limited energy output of the implant is insufficient to defibrillate the heart. If initial attempts at external defibrillation are unsuccessful, change the placement of the paddle electrodes. For example, if the sternum/apex position fails, try the anterior/posterior position.

NOTES

◯ **DRESSLER'S SYNDROME**

A pronounced form of pericarditis that develops in some patients weeks or months after an MI, characterized by pleuritic chest pain, fever, pericardial friction rub, and mild to moderate pleural effusion. The syndrome is rarely serious, though it often recurs several times before finally resolving spontaneously.

◯ **EDEMA GRADING SCALE**

Pitting >1 inch	= 4+
Pitting $\frac{1}{2}$ to 1 inch	= 3+
Pitting $\frac{1}{4}$ to $\frac{1}{2}$ inch	= 2+
Pitting <$\frac{1}{4}$ inch	= 1+

◯ **EINTHOVEN'S TRIANGLE** (see EKG Lead Placement)

◯ **EJECTION FRACTION**

First-pass angiocardiography is used to show end-diastolic and end-systolic images, shunts, and details of heart wall motion. From these values, an ejection fraction (EF) can be determined, indicating the percentage of ventricular chamber emptying. It is determined by this formula: subtract the end-systolic volume (ESV) from the end-diastolic volume (EDV), divide the result by the EDV, and multiply by 100:

$$EF = \frac{EDV - ESV}{EDV} \times 100$$

Normal ejection fraction is 60% to 65% (±8%); lower values indicate ventricular dysfunction, whereas an ejection fraction of less than 35% indicates serious ventricular problems.

NOTES

● EKG: ABERRANCY VERSUS ECTOPY (see also Ashman's Phenomenon, Dressler's Syndrome, Premature Ventricular Contractions)

RBBB Pattern

		Favors	Odds
rsR' pattern in V_1		Aberration	10:1
qRs in V_6		Aberration	20:1
R or qR in V_1 with taller left rabbit ear		L V Ectopy	10:1
QS in V_6		Ectopy	20:1
rS in V_6		L V Ectopy	7:3

LBBB Pattern

In leads V_1 or V_2:
Wide R,
slurred downstroke,
>.06 sec to nadir of S

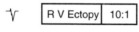

	R V Ectopy	10:1

FIGURE 2-16 Morphologic clues: ventricular aberration versus ectopy. (Adapted from Woods, S.L., Froelicher, E.S., Halpenny, C.J., & Motzer, S.U. [1995]. *Cardiac nursing* [3rd ed]. Philadelphia: J.B. Lippincott.)

● EKG: FUSION BEATS

Fusion beats occur when two opposing electrical currents meet and collide within the same chamber at the same time. The ensuing EKG complex is often narrower and of lesser amplitude than an ectopic beat alone.

REMEMBER, **with a fusion beat:** the P to P is regular, the R to R is regular, and the P **does** bear a relationship to the QRS (the PR interval may be shorter than that of the sinus rhythm, but never by more than 0.06).

NOTES

⬤ EKG: INTERPRETATION PARAMETERS (see also Myocardial Infarction: EKG Patterns)

TABLE 2-1. EKG Interpretation Parameters

Rhythm	P Wave	PR Interval	QRS Rate & Rhythm	Comment
Sinus	Before each QRS.	0.12 to 0.20	60–100. Regular.	
Sinus arrhythmia	Before each QRS.	0.12 to 0.20	60–100. Phasic variation with respiration.	
Sinus bradycardia	Before each QRS.	0.12 to 0.20	Less than 60. Regular.	Not often below 40.
Sinus tachycardia	Before each QRS.	0.12 to 0.20	Greater than 100. Regular, but may vary a little.	Usually 100–160. May be higher in children.
Sinus arrest		Pause does not march out.		R–R regular except for missed beat.
Sinus block		Pause marches out.		2nd or 3rd degree may follow.
Wandering pacemaker	Morphology changes. May be hard to see.	Varies as site changes.		R–R varies as site changes.
Premature atrial contraction (PAC)	Premature P may have different configuration. P may be buried in T.	May be less than 0.12 or more than 0.20	QRS may be normal or widened. Irregular.	No compensatory pause, usually. Frequent PACs can lead to A fib.
Premature atrial tachycardia (PAT)	Before each QRS. May be buried in preceding T wave or fused P & T.	May be less than 0.12 or more than 0.20.	160–250. Absolutely regular, usually.	QRS normal, usually. Abrupt onset and termination. Carotid pressure may terminate attack.
Atrial flutter	200–300. Sawtooth baseline.	Constant or variable.	75–300, depending on amount of AV block. Regular or irregular.	Carotid pressure produces temporary slowing, if any.
Atrial fibrillation (A Fib)	300 or more. Irregular, undulant baseline ("F" waves).	Variable. R → R never march out. Exception: CHB.	50–250, depending on degree of AV block. Irregular.	"F" waves may be shown better in V_2 than lead II. Watch for emboli.
PJC		Single premature beat interrupts rhythm. Slight delay before next.		

(continued)

TABLE 2-1. **EKG Interpretation Parameters** (Continued)

Rhythm	P Wave	PR Interval	QRS Rate & Rhythm	Comment
Junctional	Before, after, or in QRS.	40–100		
Premature ventricular contraction (PVC)	None preceding the premature QRS.		Usually normal, can occur at any rate.	Compensatory pause, usually. QRS configuration different, more than 0.12, usually.
Ventricular tachycardia (V tach)	Usually not seen. If present, are not related to QRS.	Variable.	100–220, usually. Regular or nearly regular.	QRS broad, different, more than 0.10, usually.
Ventricular fibrillation (V fib)	None.		No well-defined QRS complexes.	No palpable pulse and no audible tones.
1st degree AV block	Before each QRS.	0.21 or more.	Regular.	May be a warning that 2nd or 3rd degree block will follow.
2nd degree AV block (Type I, Mobitz I, or Wenckebach)	Before each QRS except for blocked P.	Lengthens until one beat is dropped. First of the PR series is usually >0.20 sec.	Normal.	"Group beating" is obvious. Usually a transient rhythm.
2nd degree AV block (Type II or Mobitz II)	Before each QRS except for blocked P.	Normal or prolonged but constant.	Normal if block is at bundle of HIS, wide if at the level of the bundle branches.	Is often irreversible and progresses into 3rd degree. May need pacemaker. *REMEMBER:* "Out of the blue, Mobitz II drops a Q (wave)."
3rd degree AV block (complete heart block)	Occur regularly but without relationship to QRS.	Variable	Below 60, usually. Regular, usually.	Spells of syncope common (Adams-Stokes attacks). Pacemaker is in the ventricles (idioventricular rhythm).

● EKG LEAD PLACEMENT

Most hard-wire systems utilize either five lead wires or three lead wires.

The *five-lead-wire system* allows patients to be monitored in any one of the standard 12 leads (lead I, II, III, aVR, aVL, aVF and leads V_1 thru V_6) by using the lead select on the monitor.

Position:

RA (white electrode) below right clavicle, 2nd ICS, right midclavicular line

RL (green electrode) right lower rib cage, 8th ICS, right midclavicular line

LA (black electrode) below left clavicle, 2nd ICS, left midclavicular line

LL (red electrode) left lower rib cage, 8th ICS, left midclavicular line

Chest (brown electrode) any V lead position, usually V_1 (4th ICS, right sternal border)

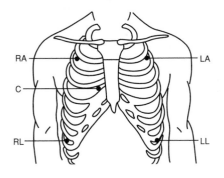

FIGURE 2-17 Five-lead-wire system. RE-MEMBER: For a quick setup—**Clouds over grass** (white electrode above green electrode) and **smoke over fire** (black electrode above red electrode).

(continued)

NOTES

The *three-lead-wire monitoring system* facilitates monitoring of the patient in any of the limb leads (lead I, II, III, aVR, aVL, aVF) by turning the lead select on the monitor.

Position:

RA (white electrode) below right clavicle, 2nd ICS, midclavicular line
LA (black electrode) below left clavicle, 2nd ICS, midclavicular line
LL (red electrode) left lower rib cage, 8th ICS, left midclavicular line

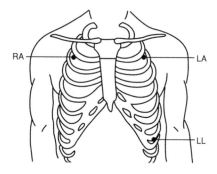

FIGURE 2-18 Three-lead-wire system. **REMEMBER:** White is right.

The chest leads are unavailable with a three-lead-wire system, but repositioning of an electrode can facilitate a modified chest lead tracing. To monitor any of the modified chest leads, the LL lead must be moved to the appropriate chest lead position, and the lead selector turned to monitor in lead III. MCL_1 and MCL_6 are the most common choices.

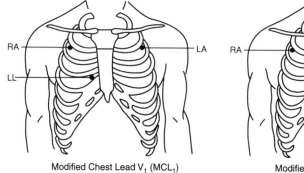
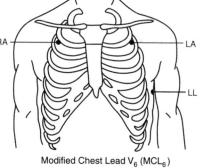

Modified Chest Lead V_1 (MCL_1)

Modified Chest Lead V_6 (MCL_6)

FIGURE 2-19 Modified chest leads.

(continued)

The *12-lead EKG* consists of viewing six leads in the frontal plane of the body and six leads in the horizontal plane at the approximate level of the 4th or 5th intercostal spaces.

TABLE 2-2. Lead Placement for 12-Lead EKG

Lead	Direction of Electrical Potential	View of Heart
STANDARD LIMB LEADS (BIPOLAR) (EINTHOVEN'S TRIANGLE)		
I	Between L arm (+) and R arm (−)	Lateral wall LV
II	Between L leg (+) and R arm (−)	Inferior wall LV
III	Between L leg (+) and L arm (−)	Inferior wall LV
AUGMENTED LIMB LEADS (UNIPOLAR)		
aVR	R arm to heart	No specific view; superior aspect LV
aVL	L arm to heart	Lateral wall; superior aspect LV
aVF	L foot to heart	Inferior wall LV
PRECORDIAL OR CHEST LEADS (UNIPOLAR)		
V_1	4th ICS; right sternal border to heart	Anteroseptal wall LV
V_2	4th ICS; left sternal border to heart	Anteroseptal wall LV
V_3	Halfway between V_2 and V_4 to heart	Anterior wall LV
V_4	5th ICS; left midclavicular line to heart	Anterior wall LV
V_5	5th ICS; left anterior axillary line to heart	Lateral wall LV
V_6	5th ICS; left midaxillary line to heart	Lateral wall LV

(continued)

NOTES

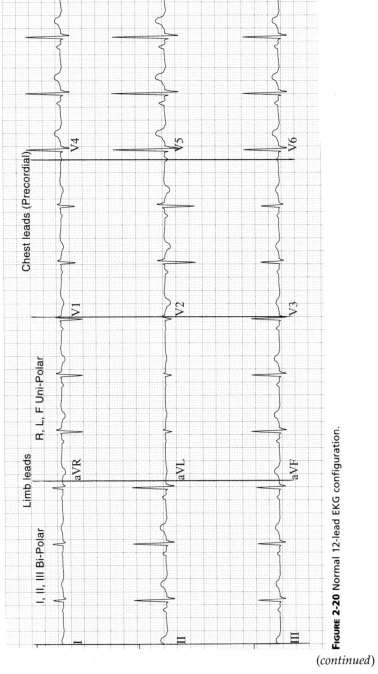

Figure 2-20 Normal 12-lead EKG configuration.

(continued)

TABLE 2-3. Normal 12-Lead EKG Waveforms

Lead	P Wave	Q Wave	R Wave	S Wave	T Wave	ST Segment
I	Upright	Small	Largest wave of complex	Small (less than R or none)	Upright	May vary from +1 to −0.5 mm
II	Upright	Small or none	Large (vertical heart)	Small (less than R or none)	Upright	May vary from +1 to −0.5 mm
III	Upright, diphasic, or inverted	Usually small or none (for large Q to be diagnostic, a Q must also be present in a VF)	None to large	None to large (horizontal heart)	Upright, diphasic, or inverted	May vary from +1 to −0.5 mm
aVR	Inverted	Small, none, or large	Small or none	Large (may be QS complex)	Inverted	May vary from +1 to −0.5 mm
aVL	Upright, diphasic, or inverted	Small, none, or large (to be diagnostic, Q must also be present in I or precordial leads)	Small, none, or large (horizontal heart)	None to large (vertical heart)	Upright, diphasic, or inverted	May vary from +1 to −0.5 mm
aVF	Upright	Small or none	Small, none, or large (vertical heart)	None to large (horizontal heart)	Upright, diphasic, or inverted	May vary from +1 to −0.5 mm
V_1	Upright, diphasic, or inverted	None or QS complex	Less than S wave or none	Large (may be QS)	Upright, diphasic, or inverted	May vary from 0 to +3 mm
V_2	Upright	None (rare QS)	Less than S wave, or none (larger than V_1)	Large (may be QS)	Upright	May vary from 0 to +3 mm
V_3	Upright	Small or none	Less, greater, or equal to S wave (larger than V_2)	Large (greater, less, or equal to R wave)	Upright	May vary from 0 to +3 mm
V_4	Upright	Small or none	Greater than S (larger than V_3)	Smaller than R; (smaller than V_3)	Upright	May vary from +1 to −0.5 mm
V_5	Upright	Small	Larger than R in V_4; less than 26 mm	Smaller than S in V_4	Upright	May vary from +1 to −0.5 mm
V_6	Upright	Small	Large; less than 26 mm	Smaller than S in V_5	Upright	May vary from +1 to −0.5 mm

U waves may follow T waves, particularly in leads V_2 to V_4; are upright; and are of lower amplitude than T waves.

(Adapted from Goldschlager, N., Goldman, M.J. (1989). *Principles of Clinical Electrocardiography,* 13th ed. Norwalk, CT: Appleton & Lange. With permission.)

◑ ENDOCARDITIS

Most common causative organisms of endocarditis are *Streptococcus viridans, Staphylococcus aureus.* Bacteria "set up housekeeping" on heart valve(s) and throw septic emboli. Mitral valve is most commonly affected; aortic valve is second. Causes related to:

- Rheumatic heart disease
- Open-heart, GU, or Gyn surgery
- Congenital heart defects
- Dental procedures
- Abscess
- Drug abuse

Assessment reveals clubbing of fingers and splinter hemorrhages of nails, petechiae, Roth's spots (white spots on retina) and Janeway lesions (painless lesions on palms, soles).

◑ ENZYMES (see Cardiac Enzymes)

◑ ERB'S POINT (see Heart Sounds: Landmarks)

◑ FEMORAL BYPASS SURGERY

- **Femoral-femoral bypass:** Performed in poor risk patients who present with unilateral claudication or ischemia. This surgery is performed only if donor artery has no marked proximal stenosis.

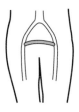

FIGURE 2-21 Femoral-femoral bypass.

(*continued*)

NOTES

- **Femoral-popliteal bypass:** Remains the standard operation for relieving ischemic symptoms secondary to femoral-popliteal occlusive disease. Patients presenting with this disease usually have involvement of distal popliteal artery and its tibial branches as well.

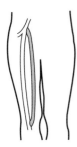

FIGURE 2-22 Femoral-popliteal bypass.

- **Aorto-iliac bypass:** Limb-threatening ischemia is not usually seen with aortoiliac occlusions unless femoral-popliteal disease is also present. Aorto-iliac occlusive disease is that in which the distal aorta, including the iliac arteries, is affected.

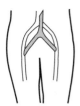

FIGURE 2-23 Aorto-iliac bypass.

- **Aorto-bifemoral bypass:** Same as aorto-iliac bypass.

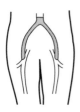

FIGURE 2-24 Aorto-bifemoral bypass.

FUSION BEATS (see EKG: Fusion Beats)

NOTES

◉ HEART SOUNDS: LANDMARKS

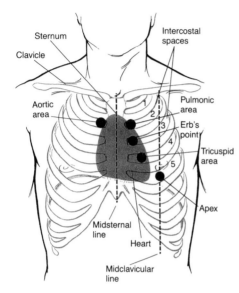

FIGURE 2-25 Locations of the auscultatory points for the various heart sounds. Note that the mitral sound is heard directly over the point of maximal impulse (PMI), which is also the apex of the heart, normally at about the midclavicular line. **REMEMBER:** Aortic on the right, pulmonic on the left, tricuspid 'neath the sternum. Mitral at the apex beat and this is how we learn 'em. (Adapted from Porth, C.M. [1994]. *Pathophysiology: Concepts of altered health states* [4th ed.]. Philadelphia: J.B. Lippincott.)

◉ HEART SOUNDS: NORMAL

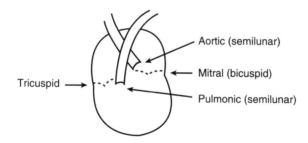

- - - - = Close for S1. (Split S1 = mitral closes before tricuspid.)
Beginning of systole.

▬▬ = Close for S2. (Split S2 = pulmonic closing before aortic. Aortic *normally* closes before pulmonic, but ear cannot distinguish this split.) End of systole, beginning of diastole.

Sequence:
S1 = Tricuspid, mitral close. (Aortic, pulmonic open.)
S2 = Aortic, pulmonic close. (Tricuspid, mitral open.)

FIGURE 2-26 Normal sequence of heart sounds.

(*continued*)

S1

S1 coincides with the R wave. Mitral and tricuspid valves close.

- Loud S1 = short PR interval (may be due to structure of AV valve, ie, mitral stenosis).

- Increased atrial pressures = valve remains open during diastole. May also be due to left to right shunting, fever, anemia, hyperthyroid.

- S1 louder after exercise.

- Soft S1 = decreased strength of contraction (due to infarct, CHF).

- If S1 of varied intensity (loud-soft-loud) may be due to atrial fibrillation or AV block.

S2

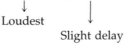

S2 sound is when the aortic and pulmonic valves close

       ↓   ↓

   Loudest

            Slight delay

 HEART SOUNDS: ABNORMAL

S3

S3 (ventricular gallop) occurs when the mitral and tricuspid valves open and there is an inrush of blood from the atria.

Sounds like KEN − TUC − KY (accent on last syllable)

        ↓   ↓   ↓

        S1   S2   S3

- Occurs on inspiration. Best if heard at beginning of expiration. Easier to auscultate if patient holds breath.

- Must use bell at lower left sternal border (left ventricular area).

- S3 can be felt; it is palpable.

- Heard in 85% of 10 to 25 year olds and is normal. Not often heard in children under 10 years old.

- Abnormal finding after 30 years of age. First subtle sign of cardiac failure, as it indicates an increase in preload (LVEDP). Can be auscultated, and S3 is heard before rales.

- If S3 persists despite diuretics and digoxin, prognosis is poor.

- S3 associated with increase in pressure and blood volume during diastole; therefore, may be heard in patient with left ventricular failure. May also be present with left to right shunt or mitral/tricuspid regurgitation.

(continued)

S4

S4 (atrial gallop) occurs when the atria contract. An inrush of blood to the ventricles sets up vibrations indicating an increased resistance to filling.

Sounds like TEN − NES − SEE (accent on first syllable)
$$\downarrow \qquad \downarrow \qquad \downarrow$$
$$\text{S4} \qquad \text{S1} \qquad \text{S2}$$

• Normal in infants, children.

• Abnormal in adults, but common in elderly.

• Usually occurs with angina; may occur with MI.

• Must use bell. Best heard at apex or left lateral sternal border. Easier to auscultate if patient holds breath.

• Indicates cardiac pathology, but not always diagnostic of a specific dysfunction.

• May be due to impairment of ability of ventricle to distend (eg, after MI) or due to increased ventricular pressure (aortic stenosis or hypertension).

Guidelines to help differentiate a left-sided gallop from a right-sided gallop:

• Left-sided gallop sounds are best heard in the apical area, while right-sided sounds are best heard at the lower left sternal border.

• The history and the suspected underlying cause of the gallop gives a clue to whether it is caused by the right or left side.

• Start at the apex and inch your way to the lower left sternal border. A left-sided gallop fades as you near the sternal border. If the gallop is from the right side, it becomes louder as you near the lower left sternal border area.

• Right-sided gallops are often heard best at the end of inspiration.

• Left-sided gallops are often heard best during expiration.

Split S1

Split S1 occurs when the mitral valve closes **before** the tricuspid.

• Occurs with right bundle branch block and PVCs.

• Heard best at the 4th left intercostal space (right ventricular area), lower left sternal border.

• Heard on expiration.

Split S2

Split S2 is physiologic. The aortic valve **normally** closes before the pulmonic, but the ear usually cannot distinguish the split.

(continued)

• Heard **only** during inspiration at pulmonic area and Erb's point (2nd or 3rd left intercostal space, adjacent to the sternum).

• After age 50, split not usually heard (aortic component delayed and valves closing closer in time).

• Fixed split occurs on inspiration **and** expiration. May occur with right bundle branch block (due to lots of blood back into the right ventricle, ie, ventricular septal defect, pulmonic insufficiency, etc).

• Reverse split is due to a delay in aortic valve closure. It is caused by blood overload in the left ventricle due to aortic stenosis, left bundle branch block, or ischemia in the left ventricle. It is heard on expiration (as aortic and pulmonic valves fuse on inspiration).

Guidelines to help differentiate a split S2 from an S3:

• When listening for an S3, be sure to use bell.

• Have patient lie in the left lateral position.

• If a split S2 is suspected, press down firmly on the bell. If it is a low-frequency gallop sound, it usually disappears. But if it is a split S2, the sound can still be heard.

• If a split S2 is suspected, inch your way up from the apex to the base (to the pulmonic and aortic area); a split S2 increases in intensity and an S3 fades away.

• An S3 is low pitched, so if two high-pitched sounds are heard, it is a split S2.

Guidelines to help differentiate a split S1 from an S4:

• When listening for an S4, be sure to use bell.

• Have patient lie in the left lateral position.

• If a split S1 is suspected, press down firmly on the bell. If it is a low-frequency gallop sound, it usually disappears. If it is a split S1, the sound can still be heard.

• If a split S1 is suspected, feel for the apical pulse. If the sound occurs before the apical pulse, it is an S4. If it occurs with the apical pulse, it is a split S1.

• If you hear three sounds where an S1 should be, it is probably a split S1 with an S4.

Murmurs

Murmurs are technically not a heart sound, but related to a pathologic event. They may be due to:

• Increased velocity of blood flow (ie, anemia, hyperthyroid)

• Narrowing of vessel (plaque, tumor)

• Blood flowing **forward** to dilated area of blood vessel (aneurysm)

(continued)

- Blood flowing **forward** through abnormal valve (aortic, mitral stenosis)
- Blood flowing through a defect (intraventricular)

SYSTOLIC MURMURS
Systolic murmurs are heard between S1 and S2. The sound is produced when the ventricle contracts. They are related to mitral, tricuspid insufficiency (regurgitation) or aortic, pulmonic stenosis.

DIASTOLIC MURMURS
Diastolic murmurs are heard between S2 and S1. The sound is produced when the ventricle fills. They are related to mitral, tricuspid stenosis or aortic, pulmonic insufficiency (regurgitation).

REMEMBER this chart to help differentiate systolic and diastolic murmurs:

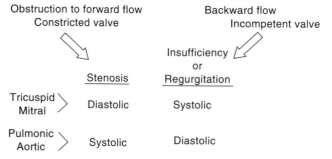

	Stenosis	Insufficiency or Regurgitation
Tricuspid Mitral	Diastolic	Systolic
Pulmonic Aortic	Systolic	Diastolic

FIGURE 2-27 Differentiating systolic from diastolic murmers.

MURMUR GRADES
Two systems are in general use for grading the intensity of murmurs: one based on four and the other on six intensities. The four-grade system is simpler and is usually adequate:

Grade 1	Faintest murmur you can hear
Grade 2	Soft
Grade 3	Loud
Grade 4	Very loud

The six-grade system is more complex, but more definitive:

Grade 1	Faintest murmur you can hear; often not heard at first
Grade 2	Faint, but heard without difficulty
Grade 3	Soft, but louder than grade 2
Grade 4	Loud, but less than grade 5
Grade 5	Loud, but not heard if stethoscope is lifted just off chest
Grade 6	Maximum loudness; heard even if stethoscope is lifted from chest

(*continued*)

When using either of these grading systems, you must identify which criteria you are using to identify the murmur: that is, grade 2/4 murmur indicates the murmur is a grade 2 on a scale of 4, or grade 4/6 murmur indicates a grade 4 murmur on a scale of 6.

If deep inspiration changes the intensity of a murmur, this should be noted. Erb's point (3rd intercostal space, left sternal border) is usually referred to for murmurs during auscultation.

◯ HEMODYNAMICS (see Swan-Ganz: Hemodynamic)

◯ HYPOVOLEMIC SHOCK (see Shock, Hypovolemic)

◯ INTRAAORTIC BALLOON COUNTERPULSATION

Useful in cardiogenic shock, MI, and postop support to:

1. Increase cardiac output

2. Decrease myocardial O_2 consumption

3. Increase aortic pressure

4. Decrease afterload (SVR)

Contraindications:

1. Incompetent aortic valve

2. Chronic end-stage heart disease

3. Peripheral vascular disease

4. Dissecting aortic or thoracic aneurysm

5. Irreversible brain damage

(continued)

NOTES

On X-ray film, tip of balloon should be at the 2nd or 3rd intercostal space, 1 to 2 cm from the left subclavian and above the renal arteries.

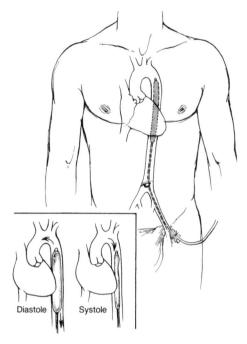

Diastole   Systole

FIGURE 2-28 Intra-aortic balloon placement.

Any of three signals, (1) EKG; (2) arterial wave; or (3) intrinsic (internal) pump rate, can trigger the pump, but the *preferred signal is the EKG,* which triggers off the R wave. The pump is initially set to inflate the balloon in the middle of the T wave (diastole) and deflate just prior to the QRS complex (systole). An appropriately sized EKG signal must be transmitted to the balloon pump to initiate pumping.

The *arterial waveform can be used as an alternative to EKG triggering* if an inconsistent EKG trigger occurs. During arterial triggering, the pump is activated by the upstroke of the arterial wave; thus, a steep upstroke is necessary, and the pulse pressure must be at least 20 mmHg.

The *internal trigger* is used only when the patient has no inherent heart rhythm and CPR does not produce a pulse, or when the patient is coming off of cardiopulmonary bypass.

Timing

The balloon should be set to inflate at the dicrotic notch (beginning of diastole when the aortic valve closes). The U shape of the patient's unassisted beat should change to a V shape when properly set. The balloon should be set to deflate at the end of diastole, during isovolumetric contraction, just prior to the opening of the aortic valve.

(continued)

REMEMBER these six key points to setting IABP timing:

1. Inflation at dicrotic notch

2. Crisp "V" shape on inflation

3. Peak *diastolic* pressure (PDP) **greater than** peak *systolic* pressure (PSP)

4. Crisp "V" shape on deflation

5. *Balloon* aortic end diastolic pressure (BAEDP) **less than** *patient's* aortic end diastolic pressure (PAEDP) (by 5 to 15 mmHg)

6. *Assisted peak* systolic pressure (APSP) **less than** *peak* systolic pressure

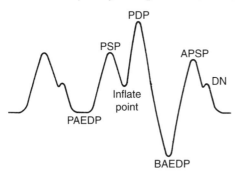

FIGURE 2-29 Correct intra-aortic balloon pump timing. (Adapted from Hudak, C.M., Gallo, B.M., & Morton, P.B. [1998]. *Critical care nursing* [7th ed.]. Philadelphia: Lippincott-Raven.)

The first three key points refer to inflation:

1. The inflation point should be at or slightly above (within 2 mm) the level of the dicrotic notch (DN).

2. The shape should be a crisp "V," showing timely inflation to maximize effect.

3. The peak diastolic pressure reflects an increase in diastolic pressure and coronary artery perfusion pressure. It should be greater than the peak systolic pressure.

The last three key points refer to deflation:

4. The crisp "V" indicates proper diastolic unloading.

5. The balloon assisted end diastolic pressure should be 5-15 mm lower than the patient's own end diastolic pressure, producing a lower pressure for the subsequent ventricular systole.

6. Compare systolic pressures. Systolic pressure after an augmented beat (APSP) should be decreased from the patient's own systolic pressure, reflecting the effect of unloading.

REMEMBER: The IABP must be set on a **2:1 augmentation** to assess timing. 1:1 or 1:3 augmentation can be initiated per order after timing has been optimized.

(continued)

TIMING ERRORS

Early inflation (inflation of the IAB prior to aortic valve closure) causes potential premature closure of the aortic valve. This can also cause a potential increase in LVEDV and LVEDP as well as an increase in the PCWP. It increases the stress on the left ventricular wall resulting in an increased afterload and an increased M$\dot{V}O_2$ demand. The waveform will show inflation prior to the dicrotic notch, and diastolic augmentation will fade onto systole.

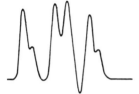

FIGURE 2-30 Early inflation.

Late inflation (inflation of the IAB markedly after the closure of the aortic valve) results in suboptimal coronary artery perfusion. The waveform shows inflation late after the dicrotic notch and an absence of a sharp V form.

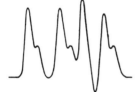

FIGURE 2-31 Late inflation.

Early deflation (premature deflation of the IAB during the diastolic phase) not only causes suboptimal coronary artery perfusion, but it sets up a potential for retrograde coronary and carotid blood flow, resulting in angina (and increased M$\dot{V}O_2$ demand). The waveform will show a sharp drop following diastolic augmentation, and assisted aortic end-diastolic pressure may be equal to or greater than the patient's own aortic end-diastolic pressure. Assisted systolic pressure may also rise.

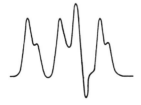

FIGURE 2-32 Early deflation.

(continued)

Late deflation (premature deflation of the IAB late in the diastolic phase, as the aortic valve is beginning to open) negates the opportunity for any afterload reduction. There is an increase in $M\dot{V}O_2$ consumption due to the left ventricle ejecting against a greater resistance and a prolonged isovolumetric contraction phase. In fact, the late deflation of the IAB may impede left ventricular ejection and may actually increase afterload. The waveform will show the assisted aortic end-diastolic pressure and the patient's own aortic end-diastolic pressure as equal. The rate of rise of the assisted systole is prolonged, and diastolic augmentation may appear widened.

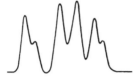

Figure 2-33 Late deflation.

REMEMBER: The worst timing errors are **early inflate** and **late deflate**, as both increase the afterload (whereas late inflate or early deflate only reduce coronary artery filling). Keep good etiquette in mind; **do not come to the party too early, or stay too late!**

IABP Weaning Criteria

- Cardiac index $>2L/min/m^2$
- PCWP <18 to 20 mmHg
- SBP >100 mmHg
- Urine output >30cc/hr
- Absence of crackles, no S3
- Improved mentation
- Absence of life-threatening dysrhythmias
- Absence of ischemia on EKG
- HR <100 bpm

NOTES

⦿ INTRAARTERIAL PRESSURE (see also Mean Arterial Pressure)

There are four characteristics inherent to an adequate arterial pressure line tracing:

1. Initial sharp rise

2. Rounded tip

3. Dicrotic notch

4. Tapering off of downstroke after dicrotic notch

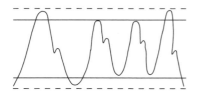

FIGURE 2-34 Normal intra-arterial pressure waveform.

The dicrotic notch is the first notch above diastole. If there is a "fling" or "whip" in the catheter, a false dicrotic notch may be produced resulting in erroneously high readings.

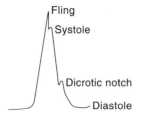

FIGURE 2-35 Arterial line catheter "fling." (DeGroot, K. [1986]. Monitoring intra-arterial pressure. *Critical Care Nurse, 6 [1].* Reprinted with permission.)

Hypovolemia results in an undulating baseline with respirations, and therefore a lowered dicrotic notch (caused by delay in closing of the aortic valve, resulting from prolonged filling time).

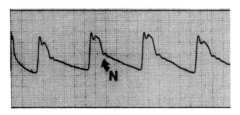

FIGURE 2-36 Arterial line tracing in a patient with hypovolemia. (DeGroot, K., Damato, M. [1986]. Monitoring intraarterial pressure. *Critical Care Nurse, 6 [1].* Reprinted with permission.)

Arterial line pressure may be **higher than cuff pressures,** and a disparity of **5 to 20 mmHg** is acceptable. However, if the cuff pressure is ever higher than the arterial line pressure, there is probably equipment malfunction or a technical error.

○ **LEAD PLACEMENT** (see EKG Lead Placement)

○ **LOWN-GANONG-LEVINE SYNDROME** (see also Wolff-Parkinson-White Syndrome)

The Lown-Ganong-Levine syndrome is a variation of the WPW preexcitation syndrome in which accessory fibers are utilized and the septum stimulated too early. The pathway associated with this syndrome is thought to join with the atria and bundle of HIS (rather than with the ventricular myocardium). Thus, the normal impulse from the sinus node can bypass the slow AV conduction. As with WPW, reciprocating tachyarrhythmias can easily occur, and management is directed at same.

Hallmarks of LGL syndrome:

• Normal rate, rhythm, and QRS

• PR interval short (<0.12 sec) with a tendency to PVST, atrial fibrillation, or atrial flutter

○ **MEAN ARTERIAL PRESSURE** (see also Intraarterial Pressure)

Normal is 70 to 110 mmHg. To calculate, *REMEMBER* **1, 2, 3**: systolic BP plus (diastolic BP × 2), divided by 3.

$$\frac{\text{systolic BP} + (\text{diastolic BP} \times 2)}{3}$$

○ **MYOCARDIAL INFARCTION: EKG PATTERNS**

Lateral

▪ **Blockage:** Circumflex branch of left anterior descending.

▪ **EKG patterns:** I, aVL, V_5, V_6 with abnormal Q wave; ST elevation; T wave inversion.

▪ **Watch for:** Transient heart blocks (may require temporary pacing).

Inferior

▪ **Blockage:** Right coronary artery.

▪ **EKG patterns:** II, III, aVF with abnormal Q wave; ST elevation; T wave inversion.

▪ **Watch for:** Transient AV blocks, usually Wenckebach block. May require temporary pacing, but rarely is a permanent pacer needed. Watch for right ventricular failure (JVD, hepatojugular reflex, increased CVP, peripheral edema). Check for new systolic murmur (papillary muscle rupture).

(continued)

Anterior

- **Blockage:** Left anterior descending artery.
- **EKG patterns:** I, aVL, V_1 through V_4 with abnormal Q wave; loss of R wave progression; ST elevation; T wave inversion.
- **Watch for:** Right bundle branch block, Mobitz type II block (indication for permanent pacemaker). Once a block develops, if a significant amount of the anterior wall is damaged, there is a good chance complete heart block will follow. If greater than 50% of the ventricle is damaged, the patient can go into cardiogenic shock with a mortality rate of >85%. Check for a new systolic murmur (ventral/septal defect or ventricular aneurysm).

Posterior

- **Blockage:** Right coronary artery, circumflex.
- **EKG patterns:** No leads view the posterior surface directly, therefore this MI is diagnosed on the basis of reciprocal EKG changes occurring in leads V_1 and V_2 (just the opposite of an anterior wall MI). Tall R wave (rather than a Q wave), ST depression (rather than elevation), and tall symmetrical T wave.
- **Watch for:** Same complications as for inferior, though not as severe.

Septal

- **Blockage:** Septum.
- **EKG patterns:** V_1 to V_2 possible changes to Q, ST, T.

Anterolateral

- **Blockage:** Left anterior descending and circumflex.
- **EKG patterns:** I, aVL, V_1 through V_6 possible changes to Q, ST, T.

Anteroseptal

- **Blockage:** Left anterior descending.
- **EKG patterns:** V_1 through V_4 possible changes to Q, ST, T. Loss of septal R wave in V_1.

Subendocardial

- **Blockage:** Nontransmural.
- **EKG patterns:** No pathologic Q wave, some loss of R wave, depressed ST segment, deep symmetrical T wave inversion.

Right Ventricular

- **Blockage:** Right coronary artery.
- **EKG patterns:** V_1 possible changes to Q, ST, T.

(continued)

Injury
ST-T wave elevation with reciprocal depression.

Ischemia
ST-T wave depression, T wave inversion, horizontal ST segments, tall pointed T waves, inverted U wave.

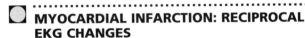

◐ MYOCARDIAL INFARCTION: RECIPROCAL EKG CHANGES

In the leads opposite the injured area, opposite (reciprocal) changes can be seen. These changes denote the extra workload to the other parts of the heart to compensate for the damaged area. There will be no Q wave, with tall upright Ts and perhaps some increase in the height of the R wave. It is impossible to determine a reciprocal change of an acute MI from ischemia, because both cause ST depression.

TABLE 2-4. Reciprocal EKG Changes in Myocardial Infarction

Primary EKG Change	Reciprocal Change
Anterior (V_1, V_2, V_3)	Inferior (II, III, aVF)
Lateral (I, aVL, V_5, V_6)	Inferior (II, III, aVF)
Inferior (II, III, aVF)	Lateral and anterior (I, aVL, V_1 to V_6)
Posterior (V_1, V_2, V_3)	Anterior (V_1, V_2, V_3)

◐ MYOCARDIAL INFARCTION: ST SEGMENT MONITORING

The ST segment is identified as occurring 60 to 80 msec after the J point in the EKG. It is the resting phase between depolarization and repolarization and is therefore isoelectric. A change in this segment usually occurs early in MI, then returns to isoelectric in minutes to hours. During coronary spasm, the ST segment elevation often precedes pain by minutes. Sustained ST elevation (3 months or longer) after an MI usually indicates ventricular aneurysm.

Lead V_5 is the preferred lead for determining elevation, followed by V_1, then V_4 or V_6. If there is a known anterior infarct, the observer must look at leads V_1 or V_2.

Conditions that alter ST segment:

Depressed	Elevated
Digitalis	Head injury
Hypothermia	Hyperthyroid
Suction	
Pericarditis	

⬛ OXYGEN CONSUMPTION (see Oxygen Consumption in Part 3, Pulmonary System)

⬛ OXYGEN DELIVERY (see Oxygen Consumption in Part 3, Pulmonary System)

⬛ PACEMAKER CODES (see also Pacemaker Modes)

With the increasing complexity of pacemakers, a coding system was developed in 1974 to help identify the various modes of pacemaker operation. The coding system itself has undergone many revisions, and today it uses five letters to sort out these functions, though many pacemakers are still identified by the original three-letter code.

Letter 1 = where pacing takes place
    V = ventricle
    A = atrium
    D = dual (atrium and ventricle)
    0 = none

Letter 2 = which event the chamber senses
    V = ventricle
    A = atrium
    D = dual (atrium and ventricle)
    0 = none

Letter 3 = response to the sensed events
    T = triggers pacing
    I = inhibits firing in response to a sensed intrinsic event
    D = dual (triggers and inhibits)
    0 = none

Letter 4 = program functions; rate modulation
    P = single programmability
    M = multiple programmability
    C = communication function (telemetry)
    R = rate modulation (pacing rate can vary, rather than being fixed)
    0 = absence of programmability or rate modulation

Letter 5 = antitachyarrhythmia function
    P = pacing stimulus can be used to convert a rapid rhythm (overdrive pacing)
    S = shock intervention for cardioversion or defibrillation
    D = dual (pacing and shock capabilities)
    0 = absence of pacing and shock capabilities

◯ PACEMAKER: EPICARDIAL WIRES

Epicardial wires are inserted during surgery, sutured on myocardial surface, and brought out through patient's chest. Atrial wires exit on the patient's right, and ventricular wires exit on the patient's left. Use a connecting cable to connect the atrial pacer wires to the atrial pacer poles of the pulse generator and the ventricular pacer wires to the ventricular pacer poles of the pulse generator. If there is a problem with sensing or capture, the wires may be reversed so that the positive pole in the atria becomes the negative pole. The wires must be encapsulated if they are not connected to a pulse generator.

◯ PACEMAKER FUNCTION: DEMAND

The demand pulse generator is the basic model and prototype for most other generations of pacemakers. If you understand the settings and principles on this model, the rationale for other models will easily follow.

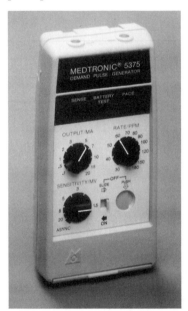

Figure 2-37 Medtronic 5375 Pacemaker, Demand. (Courtesy of Medtronic Inc., Minneapolis, MN.)

Output is in milliamps (or mA) and refers to capture. It sets the amount of voltage needed to stimulate the myocardium. Minimum energy needed for a response is called the *pacing threshold*. The mA is usually set at three times the threshold, which is normally 1.5 or less (consequently, the mA would be set at approximately 4.5). Factors that increase

(continued)

the threshold are anesthetics, acidosis, hypoxia, fibrosis on the catheter tip, low blood sugar, steroids, catecholamines, and exercise.

To measure the stimulation threshold:*

1. *Set the rate* at 10 beats *above* the patient's inherent rate to obtain 100% pacing. (Pace indicator light flashes regularly at the set rate.)

2. *Decrease output (mA)* until 1:1 capture is lost. (Pace and sense indicator lights flash intermittently.)

3. *Increase the mA* until the capture is regained. This is the mA threshold. (Pacer indicator light flashes; sense indicator light stops flashing.)

4. *Reset the mA* at two to three times the threshold in step 3. (For example, if the stimulation threshold is 2.5 mA, set the output at 5.0 mA.)

5. *Don't forget* to restore pulse generator to original pacing rate.

In some institutions, RNs are not allowed to perform this function.

Sensitivity is in millivolts (mV) and determines when the pacemaker fires. Imagine a window with 1.0 mV at the bottom of it with the window barely open, and 20 mV at the top of it with the window wide open. At 1.0 mV, a QRS complex, no matter how small, cannot fit through the window without being detected. Every QRS can be seen, and a charge is delivered only when the pacer doesn't see a QRS. This is the most sensitive position and is *demand* or *synchronous pacing.* Conversely, with the sensitivity at 20 mV (and the window wide open), intrinsic QRS complexes can happen without being detected. This is the least sensitive position and is *fixed rate* or *asynchronous pacing.* The pacer fires at a fixed rate, all the time, no matter what; it doesn't care what is "going through the window."

REMEMBER: **The higher the mV setting, the less sensitive the pacing.**

To measure the sensitivity threshold:†

1. *Set the rate control* at 10 bpm *below* the patient's inherent rate; this is **contraindicated** if the patient has no intrinsic rate or if symptomatic bradycardia. (The sense indicator light flashes regularly.)

2. *Reduce the mA* to the minimum values (This avoids the risk of competitive pacing.)

3. *Turn the sensitivity control* counterclockwise (increasing the mV and making the pacemaker less sensitive) until R wave sensing is lost and the pacemaker begins firing. (The sense indicator light stops flashing, indicating a loss of sensing, and the pace indicator light starts flashing. Capture is not likely to occur at a minimum output [mA] value.)

(continued)

4. *Decrease the sensitivity value* (by decreasing the mV and making the pacemaker more sensitive) until the EKG tracing shows that sensing has been restored. (Sense indicator light starts flashing, indicating that sensing has been restored, and the pace indicator light stops flashing.) This is the sensitivity threshold.

5. *Set the mV (sensitivity)* at ½ the sensitivity threshold value obtained in step 4. (For example, if the sensitivity threshold is 5.0 mV, set the sensitivity at 2.5 mV.)

6. *Don't forget* to restore pulse generator to original pacing rate.

†In some institutions, RNs are not allowed to perform this function.

Rate is usually set at 10 bpm above the patient's intrinsic rate for demand pacing, or at 70 to 100 bpm for fixed rate pacing.

◐ PACEMAKER FUNCTION: DUAL CHAMBER

The AV sequential pacemaker is basically the same as the Demand pacemaker (see p. 94), just a bit more sophisticated. Mentally divide the pacer generator in half vertically. Think of the left side as atrial settings and the right side as ventricular settings. In AV sequential pacing, the atrial

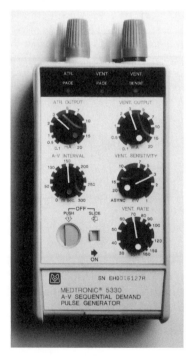

FIGURE 2-38 Medtronic 5330 Pacemaker, AV Sequential Demand. (Courtesy of Medtronic Inc., Minneapolis, MN.)

(continued)

pacing occurs at a programmed rate, regardless of any intrinsic activity, so there is no atrial sensitivity dial.

More recently, a digital AV sequential pacemaker has been developed. The same pacing principles and basic operation still apply.

Medtronic Model 5388

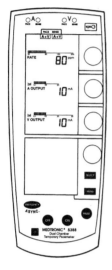
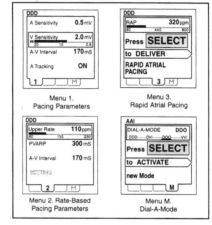

FIGURE 2-39 (Left) Medtronic 5388 Pacemaker, Dual Chamber. **(Right)** Menus for the Medtronic 5388 Pacemaker. (Courtesy of Medtronic Inc., Minneapolis, MN.)

- **To turn on:** Press ON key. Screen lights up, and dual chamber demand pacing and sensing begin at normal values.

- **To turn off:** Press OFF key twice within 5 seconds.

- **Lock/unlock:** The LOCK/UNLOCK key locks and unlocks the three upper dials. The padlock icon appears when the upper dials are locked. Use this key to unlock when adjusting the rate or output, and to relock after programming.

- **Rate and output adjustments:** After unlocking, turn rate and output dials clockwise to increase parameters and counterclockwise to decrease parameters.

- **Viewing patient's intrinsic rhythm:** Press and hold PAUSE key to suspend pacing and sensing for up to 10 seconds.

(*continued*)

- **Emergency pacing:** Press EMERGENCY to initiate high output dual chamber asynchronous pacing. Press ON key to resume pacing at current rate, output, and nominal sensitivities.
- **Menus:** Press MENU key to select one of four menus (Fig. 2-39*B*):
  Menu 1—Pacing Parameters. Adjusts atrial sensitivity, ventricular sensitivity, AV interval and atrial tracking.
  Menu 2—Rate Based Pacing Parameters. Upper rate, PVARP, and AV interval are automatically set whenever rate is adjusted, but they can be manually adjusted from this menu.
  Menu 3—Rapid Atrial Pacing. Used for overdrive pacing. **Caution:** This mode is for atrial use only. Be sure leads are connected to the atrium, and not the ventricle, before enabling.
  Menu 4—Dial-A-Mode. Allows changing pacing mode to DDD, DVI, DOO, or VVI.

PACEMAKER FUNCTION: FLEXIBLE THERAPY

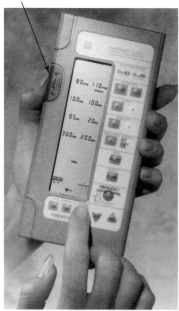

Green "press and hold" button

To turn on:
Press green "press and hold" *plus* either:
1) V PACE (for VVI)
2) MEMORY (to pace at previous setting) or
3) A-V PACE (for DDD)

To turn off:
Press green "press and hold" *plus* both green V PACE and green A-V PACE (all 3 at same time)

To change rate: press green "press and hold" button *plus* base. Rate on display should flash. Use INC or DEC arrow at bottom to change.

To change output: press green "press and hold" button *plus* either A or V. Output onscreen should flash. Use INC or DEC arrow at the bottom to change.

To view current settings: press green "press and hold" button *plus* OUTPUT, SENSITIVITY, or REFRACTORY INTERVAL. *Blue* = atrial function   *White* = ventricular function

If you lose capture: Press green "press and hold" button *plus* red EMERGENCY button. Pacer will then pace at a rate of 80, asynchronous, both chambers with maximum output (DOO).

To change mode: Press green "press and hold" button *plus* select. Use INC or DEC arrow at bottom to change.

To store parameters: After setting pacer functions, press green "press and hold." "M+" will appear in display to show there is something in memory.

FIGURE 2-40 Medtronic 5346 Pacemaker, Flexible therapy DDD function. (Courtesy of Medtronic Inc., Minneapolis, MN.)

PACEMAKER MODES

- **Atrial fixed rate (AOO) mode:** When the atria are paced but not sensed. The pacer fires at a preset rate regardless of the patient's inherent rhythm. Rarely used.

- **Ventricular fixed rate (VOO) mode:** An asynchronous, fixed rate pacing mode whereby the ventricles are paced at a preset rhythm regardless of patient's intrinsic activity and no sensing takes place.

- **Atrial demand (AAI) mode:** Used when the SA node is damaged but AV conduction is OK. In effect, it replaces the sinus impulse. The atria contract and pump blood to the ventricles causing an "atrial kick," adding 5% to 25% to cardiac output over a ventricular pacemaker. QRS complexes are the same as the intrinsic complexes.

- **Ventricular demand (VVI) mode:** Causes the ventricle to be paced, sensed, and inhibited. The pacer fires if no QRS is sensed during the preset time interval, and intrinsic cardiac activity shuts the pacemaker off. A very popular mode that is chosen 95% of the time. It is a good mode for use with atrial fibrillation with slow ventricular response and for complete heart block. The QRS complexes appear similar to right-sided PVCs.

- **AV sequential fixed rate (DOO) mode:** Paces both the atria and ventricles, but they are not sensed. The pacing is fixed and occurs at a preset rate, regardless of any inherent rhythm.

- **AV sequential (DVI) mode:** Causes the atrium to be paced at a programmed rate. Each atrial pace starts an AV interval. If there is no ventricular activity during the interval, the ventricle is paced. Atrial pacing occurs at a programmed rate, regardless of intrinsic activity (this mode does not sense P waves), and can therefore cause competitive atrial rhythms. This mode cannot be used when the patient is in atrial fibrillation or atrial flutter. Only ventricular events can be sensed and cause inhibition of the pacemaker. This mode can increase cardiac output by 20% to 50% over the cardiac output produced by ventricular pacing alone and is helpful in decreasing valve regurgitation.

- **Fully automated (DDD) mode:** Paces the atrium and ventricle, senses the atrium and ventricle, and responds to sensed events by inhibiting or triggering. When spontaneous atrial activity occurs at a rate between the programmed and upper and lower rate limits, ventricular pacing is synchronized to atrial activity. When spontaneous atrial activity occurs at a rate below the programmed lower rate limit, atrium and ventricle are paced AV sequentially. This mode is useful in patients with or without heart block, with atrial

(continued)

activity that is normal most of the time but may need backup atrial pacing periodically.

- **AV synchronous (VAT) mode:** Causes the atria to be sensed, but pacing takes place in the ventricles if no P wave is seen. If a P wave is sensed, the pacer fires simultaneously with the QRS.

TABLE 2-5. Pacemaker Mode Summary

Mode	Pace	Sense
AOO	Atrium	None
VOO	Ventricle	None
AAI	Atrium	Atrium
VVI	Ventricle	Ventricle
VAT	Ventricle	Atrium
DOO	Atrium + ventricle	None
DVI	Atrium + ventricle	Ventricle
DDD	Atrium + ventricle	Atrium + ventricle

PACEMAKER: TROUBLESHOOTING

- **No output:** Pacemaker fails to emit stimuli at programmed interval; failure to fire.
  - Battery exhaustion: Replace batteries; rule of thumb to replace every 2 to 3 days.
  - Loose set screw: Tighten screw.
  - Lead-wire fracture: Replace lead.
  - On demand, patient has inherent rate set faster than rate on pacer (pacer working correctly).
  - Pacer sensing artifact instead of inherent activity. Decrease sensitivity (counterclockwise) to make pacer more sensitive.

- **Failure to capture:** Electrical stimuli delivered by the pacemaker do not initiate depolarization of the atrium or ventricle.
  - Dislodged lead: Reposition lead; try patient on left side (electrode by gravity to ventricular wall).
  - Output too low: Increase mA.
  - Insulation break or perforation: Physician must replace lead.

- **Oversensing:** Pacemaker senses signals that should be ignored.
  - P or T wave sensing: Reduce sensitivity by increasing mA.
  - Insulation break or lead-wire fracture: Physician must replace lead.

- **Failure to sense:** Pacemaker does not start timing sequences in response to intrinsic cardiac depolarization.
  - Inadequate cardiac signal: Try patient on left side, pacer wire may be hitting septum, or adjust sensing threshold.

(continued)

• Loose set screw: Tighten screw.
• Dislodged lead: Physician must reposition.
• Insulation break or lead wire fracture: Physician must replace lead.

⬤ PATENT DUCTUS ARTERIOSUS

A normal shunting of blood from aorta to pulmonary artery occurs in a fetus and newborn, usually closing 24 to 72 hours after birth. If the closing process does not occur, the patent ductus causes a pressure load on the pulmonary circuit, resulting in right and left ventricular hypertrophy and constriction of the pulmonary arterioles. If the patent ductus is allowed to remain for many years, the pressures in the pulmonary circuit may rise to the point of becoming equal to the pressure of the systemic circuit, causing a "balanced shunt." The right-sided pressures may also exceed the left pressures, in which case there is a reversal of blood and the patient becomes cyanotic. The treatment of choice is surgical intervention.

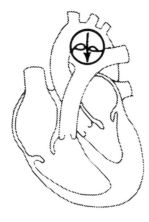

FIGURE 2-41 Patent ductus arteriosus. (Adapted from Porth, C.M. [1994]. *Pathophysiology: Concepts of altered health states* [4th ed.]. Philadelphia: J.B. Lippincott.)

⬤ PERICARDITIS

Inflammation of the pericardial sac is marked by:

1. ST elevation (then T wave inverts after ST returns to baseline)
2. Pain on inspiration, relieved by leaning forward
3. Positive heart rub
4. Positive jugular venous distension

Right and left heart pressures equalize, resulting in decreased cardiac output. Watch for tamponade. Lab work shows an increase in sedimentation rate, leukocytosis. An echocardiogram is very diagnostic.

(*continued*)

- **Pathophysiology:** Disease process → fibrin deposits → effusion (fluid in pericardial sac) → restriction → decreased diastolic filling → increased venous pressure → decreased cardiac output → decreased blood pressure.

PREMATURE VENTRICULAR CONTRACTIONS

PVCs are occasionally present in normal individuals, causing no harmful effects. They are present in 80% of patients post-MI, some being benign, and others leading to serious, even fatal, arrhythmias.

PVCs can be caused by a change in the excitability of the ventricular tissue, as induced by, for example, anesthetics, hypoxia, or digitalis; or by stimulation of the sympathetic nervous system, as induced by, for example, adrenergic drugs, emotional stress, or amphetamines.

A full compensatory pause is usually diagnostic for a PVC. The time between the beat preceding and the beat following the PVC is equal to two normal beats.

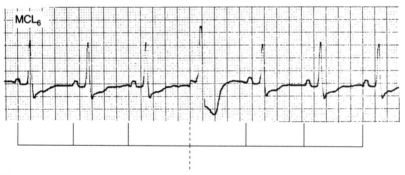

FIGURE 2-42 PVC with no interruption to sinus cycle. Lines indicate unchanged cadence. (Adapted from Woods, S.L., Froelicher, E.S., Halpenny, C.J., & Motzer, S.U. [1995]. *Cardiac nursing* [3rd ed.]. Philadelphia: J.B. Lippincott.)

(continued)

NOTES

An incomplete compensatory pause is usually diagnostic for PAC. The sinus cycle is reset.

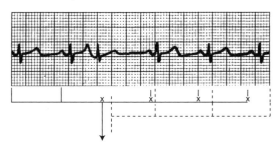

FIGURE 2-43 PAC resets sinus cycle and causes change in cadence. New regular rhythm starts at *arrow*. If old sinus cycle had been maintained, beats would fall *on dotted lines* as indicated. (Adapted from Hudak, C.M., Gallo, B.M., & Morton, P.G. [1998]. *Critical care nursing* [7th ed.]. Philadelphia: Lippincott-Raven.)

In lead MCL1, there is a 90% probability of an ectopic beat being a PVC versus an aberrancy if the left "rabbit ear" is taller than the right "rabbit ear." *REMEMBER,* the reverse is **not** true. If the left "ear" is shorter than the right "ear," it is not necessarily an aberrancy.

⬤ **PULMONARY ARTERY PRESSURES (see Swan-Ganz: Hemodynamic Normals)**

⬤ **PULMONARY CAPILLARY WEDGE PRESSURE (see Swan-Ganz: Hemodynamic Normals)**

⬤ **PULMONARY VASCULAR RESISTANCE (see Swan-Ganz: Hemodynamic Normals)**

⬤ **PULSE STRENGTH CLASSIFICATIONS**

3+ = full, bounding
2+ = normal
1+ = decreased, thready
0 = absent

◻ PULSUS ALTERNANS (see also Pulsus Paradoxus, Pulsus Magnus, Pulsus Parvus)

Alternating pulses are full and weak; that is, a strong pulse is followed by a weak pulse of equal length. Pulsus alternans is usually related to CHF.

◻ PULSUS MAGNUS (see also Pulsus Alternans, Pulsus Paradoxus, Pulsus Parvus)

Bounding pulses of pulsus magnus are usually related to thyrotoxicosis.

◻ PULSUS PARADOXUS (see also Pulsus Alternans, Pulsus Magnus, Pulsus Parvus)

Pulsus paradoxus is the absence of a pulse for >10 mmHg in arterial systolic pressure during inspiration. If pulsus paradoxus is present, the patient may be developing cardiac tamponade, shock, obstructed airway disease, constrictive pericarditis, or pulmonary embolism.

This clinical sign occurs because blood pools in the pulmonary circulation during inspiration, lowering left ventricular preload and thereby lowering cardiac output.

To determine pulsus paradoxus:

1. Place blood pressure cuff on patient and inflate above the palpated systolic pressure.

2. Slowly deflate the cuff and auscultate. The first Korotkoff sound occurs in expiration.

3. After noting the reading when the first sound occurs, continue to release the cuff pressure until sounds are audible throughout the respiratory cycle.

4. The difference between the first and second pressures is the pulsus paradoxus.

(*continued*)

NOTES

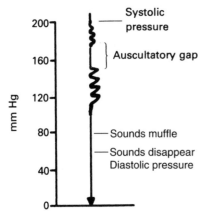

FIGURE 2-44 In pulsus paradoxus, systolic sounds are first heard at 180 mmHg. They disappear at 160 mmHg and reappear at 120 mmHg. The silent interval is the auscultatory gap. Korotkoff sounds muffle at 80 mmHg and disappear at 60 mmHg. Blood pressure is recorded as 180/80/60 with auscultatory gap. If cuff was inflated to 150 mmHg, reading may be interpreted as normotensive, when in fact patient is hypertensive. (Adapted from Bates, B. [1991]. *A guide to physical examination and history taking* [5th ed.]. Philadelphia: J.B. Lippincott.)

PULSUS PARVUS (see also Pulsus Alternans, Pulsus Magnus, Pulsus Paradoxus)

A small, weak pulse, pulsus parvus is related to aortic stenosis.

PVCs (see Premature Ventricular Contractions)

QT INTERVAL (see also Toursade du Pointe)

Normal QT interval is 0.32 to 0.40 seconds, or less than one half the preceding R to R interval.

SEPTIC SHOCK (see Shock, Septic)

NOTES

⬤ SHOCK BOX

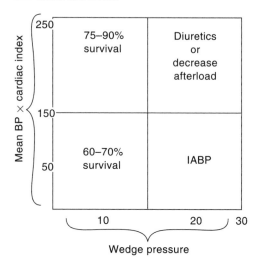

FIGURE 2-45 Shock box.

⬤ SHOCK, CARDIOGENIC

Cardiogenic shock is related to loss of myocardial contractility. *REMEMBER* **cardiogenic shock as an "engine malfunction."** It occurs mostly in MI or in conditions with deficient heart filling. What to look for:

- Increased preload (increase in CVP, PCWP, and positive JVD)
- Increased afterload (increase in SVR)
- Decreased contractility
- Decreased BP; SBP below 80 mmHg
- Decreased cardiac output

▪ **Treatment:** Fix heart muscle strength; increase contractility with positive inotropes (dobutamine, dopamine, digoxin). Decrease preload and afterload with nitroprusside (vasodilator).

⬤ SHOCK, HYPOVOLEMIC

Hypovolemic shock is related to loss of circulating blood volume. *REMEMBER* **hypovolemic shock as an "empty tank."** What to look for:

- Decreased preload (decreased CVP, PCWP)
- Increased afterload (increased SVR)
- Increased contractility
- Pulsus paradoxus
- Decreased cardiac output

▪ **Treatment:** Replace fluid loss (vasopressors contraindicated).

◯ SHOCK PARAMETERS

TABLE 2-6. Hemodynamic Parameters in Shock

Shock Type	Preload (CVP,WP)	Afterload (SVR)	Cardiac Output
Hypovolemic	↓	↑	↓
Cardiogenic	↑	↑	↓
Septic			
early	↓	↓	↑
late	↑ ↓	↑ ↓	↓
Anaphylactic	↓	↓	↓
Neurogenic	CVP ↓ WP ↑	↓	↓

◯ SHOCK, SEPTIC

Septic shock is related to bacteria (usually gram negative; rarely gram positive; often E. coli), causing massive infection (related to UTI, invasive monitoring, postpartum infections, immunosuppressant therapy, hyperalimentation, burns) and resulting in massive vasodilation. *REMEMBER* septic shock as a "tank too large."

Two stages of septic shock, each with distinct symptoms:

1. Early stage (warm, hyperdynamic):
- Warm flushed skin, chills
- Decreased urine output
- Increased respiration
- Increased cardiac output with tachycardia
- Bounding pulses
- Decreased afterload (SVR) and decreased preload (CVP, PCWP)

2. Late stage (cool, hypodynamic):
- Severe hypotension, clammy skin
- Thready peripheral pulses
- Decreased cardiac output
- Increased afterload (SVR) and increased preload (CVP, PCWP)
- Hypothermia

Treatment: Treat cause with antibiotics, steroids.

ST SEGMENT (see Myocardial Infarction: ST Segment Monitoring)

STARLING'S LAW

Starling's law states that the greater the stretch of cardiac muscle, the more forceful the heart's contraction and beat. However, when the muscle is overstretched, the force of contraction may decrease below normal level, causing circulatory failure. *REMEMBER* **a rubberband breaking when stretched too far, rendering it useless.**

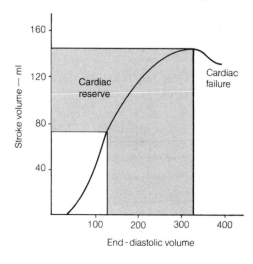

FIGURE 2-46 The Starling curve. As the end-diastolic fiber length increases so does the cardiac output. At a self-limiting end point, further stretching results in a lessened cardiac output.

STOKES-ADAMS SYNDROME

In Stokes-Adams syndrome, a syncopal episode results from inadequate cerebral blood flow, which may be accompanied by loss of consciousness as well as seizure activity. Event is precipitated by a high-grade AV block, varying periods of ventricular standstill, or asystole.

NOTES

⬤ STREPTOKINASE (see also TPA, Urokinase)

The catalyst streptokinase (Kabikinase, Streptase) converts plasminogen to plasmin and is used to treat proximal deep vein thrombosis or dissolve acute thrombi in coronary artery during MI. Streptokinase works throughout the entire body, thus the risk of local or internal hemorrhage is great. It also has been shown to produce bronchospasm, anaphylaxis, and allergic reactions. In 33% of the patients treated with streptokinase, a fever develops (treat with acetaminophen, **not** aspirin). Check for recent streptococcal infection before beginning therapy.

For administration:

1. Blood should be drawn initially, again in 4 hours, then every 12 hours (see step 5).

2. Needle sizes should be no greater than 22 gauge.

3. ABGs should be assessed only if absolutely necessary. Use radial artery with a 23 gauge needle and follow with compression for at least 30 minutes.

4. Oozing and bleeding may occur at the puncture site. Apply a pressure dressing. If oozing continues, try a pledget soaked with aminocaproic acid (Amicar).

5. Thrombin time (TT) should be 14 to 25 seconds. Monitor TT 4 hours after beginning infusion, then every 12 hours. The TT increases if the streptokinase is effective. It should be two to four times normal to achieve therapeutic action, but no greater than five times normal.

6. Observe solution for thin, translucent fibers and flocculation. These fibers can form on the outside of the drops forming an orifice, increasing the drop size and resulting in an overinfusion.

7. Streptokinase can be infused via the Swan-Ganz proximal lumen or via a central line.

See Table 2-7 for dosage.

(continued)

NOTES

TABLE 2-7. Streptokinase Dosage

Dosage Infusion Rate	Vial Content Needed	Total Volume of Solution (mL)	Pump Infusion Rate
FOR DVT:			
LOADING DOSE:			
250,000 IU/30 min	1 vial, 250,000 IU	45	90 mL/hr for 30 min
	or		
	1 vial, 750,000 IU	45	30 mL/hr for 30 min
MAINTENANCE DOSE:			
100,000 IU/hr	1 vial 750,000 IU	45	6 mL/hr
FOR MI:			
	2 vials 750,000 IU (1.5 million IU)	100	Over 30–60 min

A heparin drip should be ordered when the streptokinase infusion is complete. During therapy, there should be absolutely no new IV sites or IM meds given (use PO, NG, or existing IV lines). Monitor vital signs frequently, especially during the first hour of infusion. For emergency control of bleeding (if whole blood, PRBCs, or FFP are unavailable), use aminocaproic acid (Amicar). Usual loading dose is 5 g IVPB, then 1 g every 4 hours for 2 to 4 hours.

STROKE VOLUME

The amount of blood ejected by the heart into systemic circulation during each contraction is the stroke volume. Normal stroke volume is 60 to 130 mL/beat. It is determined by heart rate and cardiac output:

$$\frac{\text{Cardiac output}}{\text{Heart rate}}$$

STROKE VOLUME INDEX

Stroke volume index is stroke volume adjusted for individual body surface area. Normal stroke volume index is 35 to 60 mL/beat/m².

$$\frac{\text{Cardiac index}}{\text{Heart rate}} \times 1000 \quad \text{OR} \quad \frac{\text{Stroke volume}}{\text{Body surface area}}$$

S$\bar{\text{V}}$O$_2$ MONITORING (see also S$\bar{\text{V}}$O$_2$ Monitoring in Part 3, Pulmonary System)

Mixed venous oxygen saturation (S$\bar{\text{V}}$O$_2$) monitoring is performed with a fiberoptic pulmonary artery catheter that carries infrared light from the

(continued)

monitor to the distal tip of the catheter. The light from this catheter then scatters off the red blood cells it "sees," and the measurement of this is converted to a number by the monitor.

- Normal = 60% to 80%
- Below 60% for >3 min = O_2 reserve being used
- Below 50% for >3 min = O_2 reserve depleted; anaerobic metabolism (lactic acidosis begins)
- Below 30% for >3 min = O_2 reserve depleted; insufficient tissue O_2; coma

Causes of decreased $S\bar{V}O_2$:

1. Less oxygen delivered

- Fall in cardiac output (heart failure, increased afterload, increased PEEP, dysrhythmias)
- Decreased arterial saturation (suctioning, disconnect from O_2 source, respiratory failure, abnormal hemoglobin)

2. Increased oxygen demand

- Increased consumption (fever, pain, shivering, seizures, increased work of breathing, exercise)

Causes of elevated $S\bar{V}O_2$:

1. More oxygen delivered

- Rise in cardiac output (septic shock, inotropic drugs, IABP support, afterload reducing agents, thyrotoxicosis)
- Elevated arterial saturation (increases in FIO_2, hyperoxia)
- Rise in hemoglobin (polycythemia)

2. Decreased oxygen demand

- Decreased consumption (anesthesia, hypothermia, paralysis, cyanide toxicity)

Management of decreased $S\bar{V}O_2$/low cardiac output:

1. Look for correctable causes that are noncardiac (acidosis, electrolytes, respiratory)

2. Optimize preload (PCWP 15 to 18 mmHg)

3. Optimize heart rate with pacing if necessary (90 to 100 bpm)

4. Control arrhythmias

5. Assess cardiac output and start inotropes if cardiac index <2.0 L/min/m^2

6. Calculate SVR and start vasodilators if SVR >1500 dynes/sec/cm^5

7. Blood transfusions if Hct <28 to 30 g/dL

● SWAN-GANZ: CATHETER INFORMATION

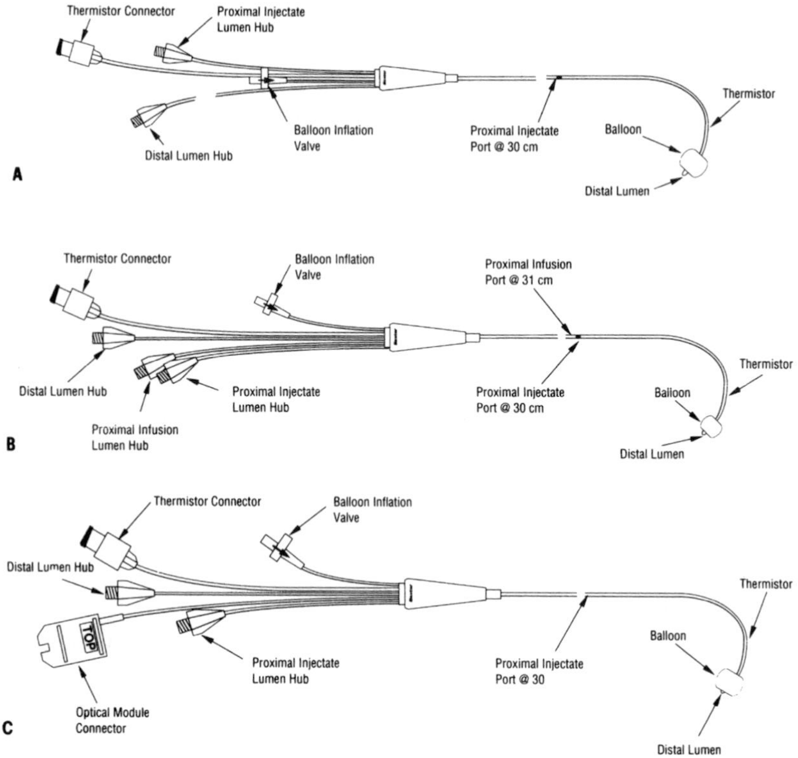

Figure 2-47 Catheter model examples. **(A)** Traditional pulmonary artery (PA) catheter. **(B)** Venous infusion port PA catheter. **(C)** Oximetry PA catheter. (*continued*)

NOTES

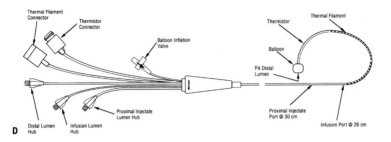

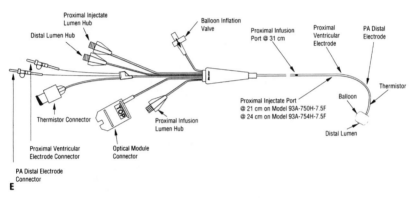

FIGURE 2-47 (CONTINUED) (D) Continuous cardiac output PA catheter. **(E)** Right ventricular ejection fraction oximetry PA catheter. (Courtesy of Baxter Healthcare Corporation, Edwards Critical-Care Division.)

- **Markings:** Fat rings = 50 cm; thin rings = 10 cm.

- **Placement:** Proximal lumen at approx. 30 cm; correct placement in right atrium. Venous infusion port (VIP) at 31 cm; superior vena cava at approx. 40 cm. Insert depth dependent on patient size; usually about 45 cm with internal jugular access.

NOTES

◐ SWAN-GANZ: HEMODYNAMIC ALGORITHM

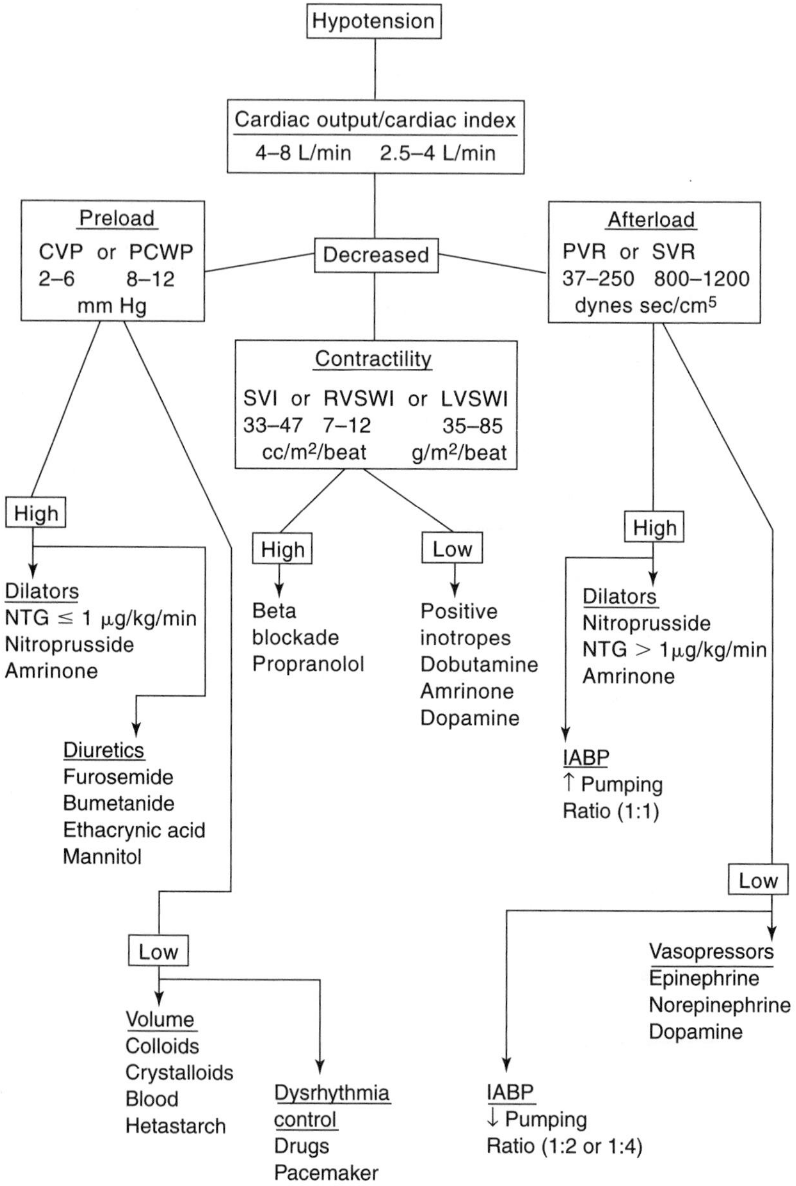

FIGURE 2-48 Hemodynamic algorithm. (Urban, N. [1986]. Integrating hemodynamic parameters with clinical decision making. *Critical care nurse, 6[2].* Reprinted with permission.)

⬤ SWAN-GANZ: HEMODYNAMIC EFFECTS OF COMMON IV MEDICATIONS

TABLE 2-8. Hemodynamic Effects of Some Common IV Medications

	HR	MAP	PAP	PWP	CVP	SVR	SV	CO
VASODILATING AGENTS								
Nitroglycerin	↑	↓	↓	↓	0/↓	↓	↑	↑
Nitroprusside	↑	↓	↓	0/↓	0/↓	↓	↑	↑
Hydralazine	↑	↓	↓	0/↓	0/↓	↓		↑
Phentolamine	↓	↓	↓	↓	↓	↓	↑	↑
VASOPRESSOR AGENTS								
Phenylephrine	0/↓	↑	↑	↑	↑	↑		↓
Metaraminol	0/↑	↑	↑	↑	↑	↑		↑/↓
MIXED ACTIVITY AGENTS								
Epinephrine	↑	↑	↑	↑	↑	↑/↓		↑
Norepinephrine	0/↑	↑	↑	↑	↑	↑		↑/↓
Ephedrine	↑	0/↑	0/↑	0/↑	0/↑	↑		↑
Dopamine	0/↑	0/↑	0/↑	0/↑	0/↑	↑		↑
INOTROPIC AGENTS								
Dobutamine	0/↑	0/↑	0	0	0/↑	0/↑		↑
Isoproterenol	↑	0/↑	0/↑	0/↓	0/↓	0/↓	↑	↑
Amrinone	0	↓	↓	↓	0/↓	↓	↑	↑
Digoxin	↓						↑	↑
ANTIARRHYTHMIC AGENTS								
Lidocaine	0	0/↓	0/↓	0	0	0/↓		0/↑
Quinidine	0/↓	↑	0/↓	0/↓	0/↑	0		↓
Procainamide	0	↓	0/↓	0/↓	0/↑	0		↓
Propranolol	↓	↓	0/↓	0/↓	0/↓	0		↓
Labetalol	↓	↓	↓	↓	↓	↓		↓
Bretylium	↑/↓	0	0	0	0	0		0
Verapamil	↑/↓	0/↓	0/↓	0/↓	0/↓	↓		↑/↓

Key: 0, little or no change; ↑, increase; ↓, decrease.
Darovic, G. (1987). *Hemodynamic Monitoring.* Philadelphia, PA: W. B. Saunders Co. Reprinted with permission.

⬤ SWAN-GANZ: HEMODYNAMIC NORMALS

Right Atrial (CVP Pressures): Normal 4 to 10 cm H₂O; 2 to 6 mmHg

Right heart filling pressures = preload (stretch). Contractility affects CVP.

Poor contractility
↓
Right atrium unable to empty completely
↓
Rise in right ventricular end-diastolic pressure
↓
Rise in CVP

(continued)

CVP increases (right ventricle can't pump volume forward) due to:
- Overinfusion of IVs (circulatory overload)
- Venous congestion (tamponade, PEEP, right ventricle failure, late left failure)
- Left to right shunt, severe mitral stenosis
- Poor contractility of right ventricle (infarct, pericarditis)
- High PVR (pulmonary edema, COPD)

CVP decreases (inadequate venous return) due to:
- Hemorrhage
- Third spacing
- Extreme vasodilation (shock)

Right Ventricle Pressures: Normal $\frac{25\text{--}30}{0\text{--}5}$ mmHg

On insertion, start recording Swan-Ganz pressures here. Keep catheter moving; an irritated ventricle causes PVCs.

Systolic pressure increases due to:
- Pulmonary hypertension
- Pulmonary stenosis

Diastolic pressure increases due to:
- Right ventricular failure
- Pericarditis
- Tamponade

Pulmonary Artery Pressures: Normal $\frac{17\text{--}32}{8\text{--}10}$ mmHg; mean <20 mmHg

Right ventricular and pulmonary artery systolic pressure should be the same, but the diastolic pressure is different.

PAP increases due to:
- Left ventricular failure
- Pulmonary vascular disease (hypertension, embolism, edema, etc)

PAP decreases due to:
- Volume depletion
- Drugs
- Aspiration
- Pulmonary stenosis

(continued)

Pulmonary Capillary Wedge Pressure: Normal 4 to 12 mmHg *

PCWP represents the pressure in the left ventricle when there is no mechanical obstruction; it correlates with pulmonary artery diastolic pressure in the absence of disease. Measure wedge pressure at end expiration. Measure at the waveform peak if the patient is not ventilated, and measure at the waveform dip if the patient is ventilated. (*REMEMBER:* **For** *ventilated* **patient, measure waveform in the** *valley*.)

*Can be normal at 14 to 18 mmHg in a compromised patient.

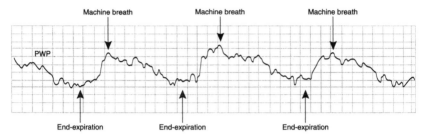

FIGURE 2-49 Pulmonary artery wedge pressure (PWP) tracing showing respiratory variation from positive pressure mechanical ventilation. In this case, PWP measurement is correctly taken at the mean point of end expiration, not in the valley.

PCWP increases due to:

• Left ventricular failure (audible S3 with increased left ventricular filling pressure)

• Tamponade

• Pulmonary edema

• Mitral stenosis or insufficiency

• Hypervolemia

PCWP decreases due to:

• Hypovolemia

• Afterload reduction caused by vasodilators

Cardiac Output (CO): Normal 4 to 7 L/min/m²

CO is the amount of blood ejected by the heart into the systemic circulation each minute.

$$CO = \text{stroke volume} \times \text{heart rate}$$

(*continued*)

CO increases due to:
- AV shunt
- Pulmonary edema
- Increased metabolic state (fever, tachycardia, burn)
- Mild hypertension with wide pulse pressure
- Early sepsis

CO decreases due to:
- PEEP (*REMEMBER:* **Peep is deep)**
- Infarct
- Decreased stroke volume (due to dehydration, diuresis, infarct, etc)
- Valve disorders
- Increased PVR
- Poor filling of left ventricle
- Hypovolemia
- Slow heart rate
- Tamponade

Cardiac Index (CI): Normal 2.5 to 4.0 L/min/m²

<1.5	grave prognosis
1.5–2.0	cardiogenic shock
2.0–2.2	onset of forward failure

Cardiac output should be adjusted for body size (see also Body Surface Area Nomogram) and is known as the cardiac index (CI).

$$CI = \text{cardiac output} \div \text{body surface area}$$

Pulmonary Vascular Resistance (PVR): Normal 37 to 250 dyne/sec/cm⁵

This provides a measurement of right ventricular afterload. PVR is the force the right ventricle must overcome to produce blood flow through the pulmonary system.

$$PVR = \frac{PAM - PCWP \times 80}{\text{Cardiac output}}$$

Pulmonary vessels constrict with a fall in the alveolar PO_2 or a rise in the arterial $PaCO_2$. An obstruction such as a pulmonary embolus can also cause the PVR to rise.

(continued)

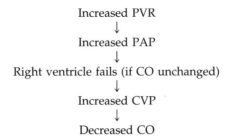

Increased PVR
↓
Increased PAP
↓
Right ventricle fails (if CO unchanged)
↓
Increased CVP
↓
Decreased CO

Systemic Vascular Resistance (SVR): Normal 800 to 1300 dyne/sec/cm^5

SVR is the resistance the left ventricle must overcome to produce blood flow. It is also known as peripheral vascular resistance (not to be confused with PVR, which is pulmonary vascular resistance and a separate entity).

A low SVR means a decreased afterload: patient is peripherally dilated.

$$SVR = \frac{MAP - CVP}{CO}$$

A high SVR means an increase in the afterload: patient is peripherally constricted.

REMEMBER: **The SVR always moves inversely to the cardiac output.**

Increased SVR can be due to:

• Hypovolemia
• Hypothermia (cold, clammy skin)
• Catecholamines
• Hypertension
• Cardiogenic shock
• Massive pulmonary embolism
• Cardiac tamponade
• Any condition causing vasoconstriction

Decreased SVR can be due to:

• Vasodilator therapy
• Early septic shock

NOTES

⬤ SWAN-GANZ: HEMODYNAMIC WAVEFORMS

A. Catheter advanced to right atrium, balloon is inflated. Pressure is low, usually 2–5 mm Hg.

B. Catheter is floated to right ventricle with the balloon inflated. Wave-forms indicate a systolic pressure of 25–30 mm Hg and a diastolic pressure of 0–5 mm Hg.

C. As the catheter moves into the pulmonary artery, the systolic pressure remains the same but the diastolic pressure elevates to 10–15 mm Hg.

D. The balloon is deflated and the catheter is moved until it can be wedged in a smaller vessel. When the balloon is inflated, the pressure recorded is that pressure in front of the catheter. It is an approximate measure of the left ventricular end diastolic pressure.

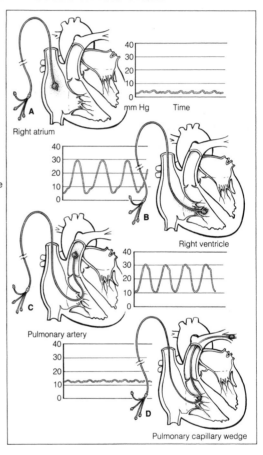

FIGURE 2-50 Insertion of a flow-directed cardiac catheter.

⬤ SWAN-GANZ: INSERTION SETUP CHECK LIST

Swan-Ganz catheter

Pressure setup, flushed (free of air and bubbles)

Sterile gowns, masks, caps, drapes, towels, gloves

Towel roll

Povidone-iodine solution (Betadine)

Sterile bowl, sterile saline for catheter flush

10-cc syringes, needles, sterile blade, suture material, transparent dressing

Sterile 4 × 4s

◻ SYSTEMIC VASCULAR RESISTANCE (see Swan-Ganz: Hemodynamic Normals)

◻ TAMPONADE

Acute compression of the heart, or tamponade, results from the collection of blood or fluid in the pericardial sac. It may occur following either blunt or penetrating chest trauma, or by bleeding into the pericardium due to the rupture of the heart or coronary vessel. Patient presents with a clinical picture of:

- Narrowing pulse pressure
- Falling systolic blood pressure
- Pulsus paradoxus >10 to 15 mmHg (see Pulsus Paradoxus)
- Distant or muffled heart sounds
- Increased preload (CVP >20 mmHg, PCWP increased)
- Widened mediastinal shadow on chest X-ray film
- Decreased cardiac output
- Cardiac pressures equalizing (RA, PAD, PCWP, LA)

Treatment consists of direct repair of the wound, a thoracotomy or pericardiotomy, or a pericardiocentesis, where an 18-gauge needle is inserted through the xiphocostal angle to aspirate the pericardial sac. Removal of as little as 10 to 20 cc may relieve the symptoms.

◻ TEE (see Transesophageal Echocardiogram)

◻ THROMBOLYTIC THERAPY (see Streptokinase, TPA, Urokinase)

◻ TISSUE PLASMINOGEN ACTIVATOR (see TPA)

NOTES

TORSADES DE POINTES

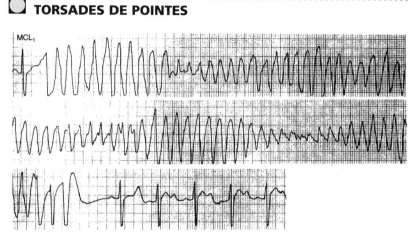

FIGURE 2-51 Torsades de pointes. Note characteristic features: (*top*) multiform QRS complexes that twist around the baseline, (*middle*) initiation by a premature ventricular complex with a long coupling interval, (*bottom*) associated long QT interval and wide TU waves during sinus rhythm.

Torsades de pointes is a dangerous form of ventricular tachycardia in which the polarity of the ventricular complexes swings between positive and negative; literally, it is a "twisting of points." The QT is prolonged, and the longer refractory period allows more ventricular ectopic contractions of various kinds. (Normal QT = 0.32 to 0.40 seconds, or less than one-half the preceding R to R interval.) Quinidine, procainamide, disopyramide, or amiodarone is usually the culprit, although anything that lengthens the QT interval could be the cause, for example, hypokalemia, hypomagnesemia, profound bradycardia, intracerebral pathology, unilateral alteration of sympathetic tone, or psychotropic drugs. The patient may be conscious, and the tachycardia may be paroxysmal, stopping and then starting again.

TPA (see also Streptokinase, Urokinase)

TPA, or tissue plasminogen activator (Alteplase or Activase), is a thrombolytic agent that converts plasminogen to plasmin at the site of the clot. TPA has a short half-life, only 2 to 5 minutes, and lytic effects last only 25 to 50 minutes. TPA is more specific than streptokinase, and therefore the risk of bleeding is less.

Criteria for use:

• Patient must be symptomatic with chest pain typical of MI for less than 6 hours in duration, preferably less than 4 hours.

(*continued*)

- Chest pain longer than 6 hours, if intermittent with ongoing signs of ischemia.
- A 1-mm ST segment elevation in two or more leads.

Preparations prior to infusion:

- Three large-bore IVs
- Initial lab work: CBC, Chem 20, PT/PTT, cardiac enzymes, liver profile, group screen, and hold
- If ABGs are required, use radial artery for puncture and avoid brachial or femoral arteries

Therapy guidelines:

- Reconstitute TPA as follows: use two 50-mg bottles added to 100 cc D5W.
- Make sure no filter is on tubing.
- Use a dedicated line.

Infusion guidelines:

- Dose is 0.5 to 1 mg per kg over 60 to 90 minutes.
- Usually given as follows: 15 cc (15 mg) IV push over 2 to 3 minutes (draw up in syringe and push).

Immediately follow with:

- 50 cc (50 mg) over 30 minutes (pump at 100 cc/hr × 30 minutes).
- 35 cc (35 mg) over 1 hour (pump at 35 cc/hr × 1 hr).

Concomitant heparin therapy:

- After TPA infusion is complete, administer 5,000 unit heparin bolus over 2 to 3 minutes.
- Begin IV heparin infusion at 1,000 U/hr.

Interventions:

- Observe for reperfusion arrhythmias and hypotension.
- Monitor coagulation profile. Watch for ecchymotic areas on patient, especially at flank.
- Avoid IM injections or arterial sticks for 24 hours.

Contraindications:

- Recent surgical procedure or GU bleeding (within 10 days)
- Recent trauma, prolonged CPR
- Diabetic or other hemorrhagic retinopathy
- Pregnancy
- Patients currently on oral anticoagulants or with uncontrolled hypertension

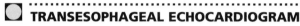

TRANSESOPHAGEAL ECHOCARDIOGRAM

An NPO status should be maintained for at least 6 hours before the study. With the patient supine or in the left lateral position, mild to moderate sedation and a local anesthetic spray to the posterior oropharynx are given. A flexible endoscope with a 2D transducer affixed to the end of it is then inserted orally and passed down the esophagus. Because of the transducers opportune position in relation to the cardiac structures, excellent images of the aorta, atria, and valves are easily obtained. While the procedure itself causes the patient little discomfort, there may be some discomfort to the chest wall following the study. Emergency equipment should always be readily available.

UROKINASE (see also Streptokinase, TPA)

Urokinase (Abbokinase) is a thrombolytic agent that acts directly on plasminogen, forming plasmin, which dissolves the clot. It is usually used for pulmonary emboli. Its half-life is 20 minutes. Rare allergic responses have been noted, and of all thrombolytic drugs, urokinase has a decreased potential for hemorrhage.

Administration:
• Via IV, 4,000 to 8,000 U/min

◯ WELLENS SYNDROME

Six warning signs proposed by Wellens are associated with critical stenosis of the proximal LAD:

1. Prior angina

2. Little or no enzyme elevation

3. No Q wave

4. Little or no ST elevation

5. ST-T turns down to negative at an angle of 60° to 90°

6. Deeply inverted symmetrical T wave

NOTES

⬤ WOLFF-PARKINSON-WHITE SYNDROME (WPW)

WPW syndrome is a ventricular "preexcitation" syndrome in which an impulse "sneaks" down a shorter path (via the Kent's bundle or the Mahaim fibers) bypassing the AV node, while at the same time, another impulse from the normal bundle of HIS pathway is conducted, resulting in the ventricle being stimulated from two directions. This sets up recurrent bouts of supraventricular tachyarrhythmias. Two types of WPW have been identified: type A on the left side of the heart and type B on the right side of the heart. The hallmarks of the syndrome are twofold: (1) a shortened PR interval (usually less than 0.12 seconds) due to the impulse taking a "short cut" from the SA to the AV node, and (2) an initial slurring on the upstroke of the QRS (delta wave), reflecting the ventricular activation outside the normal conduction system.

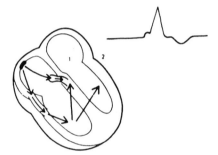

FIGURE 2-52 Wolff-Parkinson-White syndrome.

This syndrome is most often seen in young adults and rarely in the elderly. The patient can go in and out of this rhythm, exhibiting entire runs of supraventricular tachyarrhythmias or just experiencing an occasional beat or two. The syndrome may require no treatment if the occurrences are rare. However, recurrent bouts of tachyarrhythmias must be treated as appropriate with vagal maneuvers and, if they are unsuccessful, with vagotonic drugs such as digitalis. Surgical intervention to sever the Kent's bundle or Mahaim fibers bypass tract is often used for those patients who experience frequent, disabling tachyarrhythmias.

Pulmonary System

A-a GRADIENT

The A-a gradient indicates if gas transfer is normal and helps to distinguish hypoventilation from other causes. Values change with age and concentration of FIO_2, but the following rule of thumb generally applies for a young adult:

> Normal: <10 mmHg on room air
>
> >70 mmHg on 50% FIO_2

The goal is to have a decreased A-a gradient, as an increase in the gradient is usually indicative of $\dot{V}/\dot{Q}$ mismatch, shunting, and/or diffusion abnormalities.

Formula for calculation:

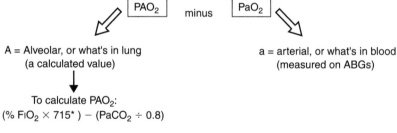

PAO_2 minus PaO_2

A = Alveolar, or what's in lung   a = arterial, or what's in blood
(a calculated value)   (measured on ABGs)

To calculate PAO_2:
$$(\% \; FIO_2 \times 715^*) - (PaCO_2 \div 0.8)$$

Example:
Patient on 70% FIO_2. $PaCO_2$ on ABGs = 35
$(.70 \times 715) - (35 \div 0.8) = \mathbf{457}$ Patient's ABG PaO_2 value = **80** mmHg

Entire equation then:
457 − 80 = 357 A-a gradient

* Equation presumes barometric pressure at sea level

Figure 3-1 A-a gradient calculation.

(continued)

REMEMBER: A quick method for approximation of this value is:

$$F_IO_2 \times 6 \times 100$$
(In the above case: $0.70 \times 6 \times 100 = 420$)

⬤ ABGs

TABLE 3-1. ABG Interpretation			
	PH 7.35–7.45	**PaCO$_2$** 35–45	**HCO$_3$** 22–26
Respiratory alkalosis	↑	↓	—
Respiratory acidosis	↓	↑	—
Metabolic alkalosis	↑	—	↑
Metabolic acidosis	↓	—	↓

Interpretation:

1. Check the pH.

   a. ↑ = alkalosis

   b. ↓ = acidosis

   c. Normal = no imbalance

2. Check the PaCO$_2$.

   a. ↑ = CO$_2$ retention (indicates hypoventilation, an increase in CO$_2$ productivity, or an increase in physiologic dead space in the setting of limited pulmonary reserve or CMV ventilator setting)

   b. ↓ = CO$_2$ blown off (indicates hyperventilation, respiratory alkalosis, or compensation for metabolic acidosis)

   c. Normal = no imbalance of respiratory component

3. Check the HCO$_3^-$.

   a. ↑ = nonvolatile acid is lost; HCO$_3^-$ is gained (indicates metabolic alkalosis or compensation for respiratory acidosis)

   b. ↓ = nonvolatile acid is added; HCO$_3^-$ is lost (indicates metabolic acidosis or compensation for respiratory alkalosis)

4. Determine the imbalance.

5. Determine if compensation exists.

REMEMBER:

   a. pH, PaCO$_2$ **opposite** direction = respiratory problem

   b. pH, HCO$_3^-$ **same** direction = metabolic problem

   c. HCO$_3^-$, PaCO$_2$ **same** direction = compensation for abnormal pH

   d. HCO$_3^-$, PaCO$_2$ **opposite** direction = 2 mixed imbalances present

(*continued*)

Respiratory Acidosis (↓ pH, ↑ PaCO₂)

Respiratory acidosis is related to stroke, drug overdose, aspiration, pneumonia, ARDS, cardiac arrest, COPD, hypoventilation, neuromuscular disorders.

- **Treatment:** Aggressive chest PT, suction. Increase respiratory rate, increase tidal volume.

Respiratory Alkalosis (↑ pH, ↓ PaCO₂)

Respiratory alkalosis is related to anxiety, fear, head trauma, brain tumor, hepatic insufficiency, fever, mechanical overventilation, pulmonary embolism, thyrotoxicosis.

- **Treatment:** Sedation, support, breathe in paper bag for attack of hyperventilation. Decrease respiratory rate, decrease tidal volume.

Metabolic Acidosis (↓ pH, ↑ HCO₃⁻)

Metabolic acidosis is related to renal failure, diarrhea, TPN, acetazolamide (Diamox) (diuretic that prevents carbonic acid formation), ketoacidosis, lactic acidosis (caused by bicarbonate loss or excess acids in extracellular fluid).

- **Treatment:** Treat underlying cause; monitor I/O and dysrhythmias; protect against infection.

Metabolic Alkalosis (↑ pH, ↓ HCO₃⁻)

Metabolic alkalosis is related to volume depletion (loss of H^+, Cl^-, K^+ from vomiting or diarrhea, gastric suction, or diuretic therapy).

REMEMBER: al-K⁺-**low**-sis means potassium value is **low** when patient is alkalotic.

- **Treatment:** Treat underlying cause; monitor I/O; potassium replacement therapy.

○ ABGs, MIXED VENOUS (see Mixed Venous ABGs)

○ ACUTE RESPIRATORY FAILURE

Defined by:

pH	↓ 7.3
PaCO₂	↑ 50–55 mmHg
PO₂	↓ 70 mmHg on 50% O₂ mask
Tachypnea	↑ 35 breaths/minute
Vital capacity	↓ 15 mL/kg
Inspiratory force	↓ 25 cm H₂O

● ALBUTEROL (see Respiratory Inhalation Medications)

● ALUPENT (see Respiratory Inhalation Medications)

● AMINOPHYLLINE

A smooth muscle relaxant, aminophylline is useful in asthma and bronchospasms.

- **IV continuous infusion:** (If patient is not chronically maintained on theophylline, an IV loading dose of 5.6 mg/kg over 30 minutes is required.) Mix 500 mg in 500 cc D5W or 0.9 NS. Titrate to therapeutic level of 10 to 20 μg/mL.

    Maintenance dose:

Adult, heavy smoker, 16–50 years	0.7 mg/kg/hr (max 0.9 mg/kg/hr)
Adult, nonsmoker >16 years	0.4 mg/kg/hr
Adult with cardiac decompensation, cor pulmonale, or liver dysfunction	0.2 mg/kg/hr

● ANATOMY, PULMONARY

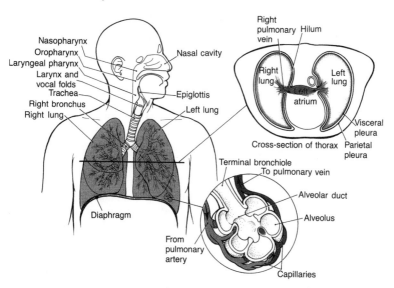

FIGURE 3-2 The respiratory system showing the upper and lower respiratory tracts. *Insets* show the alveoli and a horizontal cross-section of the lungs.

(continued)

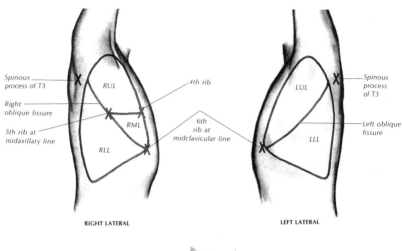

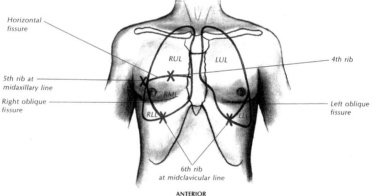

FIGURE 3-3 Location of lung lobes.

⬤ ANION GAP

It is normal to have approximately the same number of anions and cations circulating in the blood; however, because there are a certain number of them that are not routinely measured, a "gap" exists, with normal ranging from 8 to 16 mEq/L. The formula to calculate the anion gap is:

$$Na^+ - (Cl^- + HCO_3^-)$$

A calculated anion gap of more than 16 mEq/L indicates there is an increase in the number of unmeasured anions (which has decreased the number of measured anions). Because most unmeasured anions are acids (lactate, ketone bodies, poisons), the gap usually results in metabolic

(continued)

acidosis, although other forms of acidosis may also produce increases in the gap.

Decreases in the anion gap are rare, though their clinical significance is equally important.

TABLE 3-2. Causes of Altered Anion Gap
● ●

■ **INCREASED ANION GAP**

INCREASED UNMEASURED ANIONS
Endogenous metabolic acidosis
　Lactic acidosis
　Ketoacidosis
　Uremic acidosis
Exogenous anion ingestion
　Ethylene glycol
　Methanol
　Paraldehyde
　Salicylates
　Penicillin
　Carbenicillin
Increased plasma proteins
　Hyperalbuminemia

DECREASED UNMEASURED CATIONS
Hypokalemia
Hypocalcemia
Hypomagnesemia

■ **DECREASED ANION GAP**

INCREASED UNMEASURED CATIONS
Normal cations
　Hypercalcemia
　Hyperkalemia
　Hypermagnesemia
Abnormal cations
　Increased globulins (eg, myeloma)
　Lithium

DECREASED UNMEASURED ANIONS
Hypoalbuminemia

● ●
■ **ARDS (Shock Lung, Liver Lung)**

Adult respiratory distress syndrome (ARDS) is a form of noncardiogenic pulmonary edema that can cause acute respiratory failure. It usually results from an indirect injury to the lungs, from shock, sepsis, DIC, or

(continued)

pancreatitis, or from a direct injury such as near-drowning, aspiration, pneumonia, or chest trauma. By definition, ARDS is:

1. Three or four quadrant alveolar filling

2. Compliance less than 40 cc/cm H_2O

3. PaO_2/FiO_2 less than 150

4. Pulmonary artery wedge pressure less than 18 mmHg

The signs and symptoms are subtle: high peak inspiratory pressures, increase in the A-a gradient, decreased compliance, decreased functional residual capacity, and hypoxia (even with 100% oxygen and high ventilation pressures). A "ground glass" appearance on chest X-ray is common. The treatment goal is to increase the functional residual capacity, usually with the assistance of PEEP (after assessing for hypovolemia) and fluid restriction.

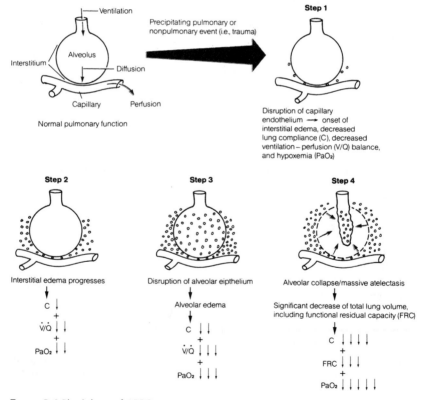

FIGURE 3-4 Physiology of ARDS.

ARTERIAL BLOOD GASES (see ABGs)

ARTERIAL O₂ CONTENT

Arterial oxygen content, or CaO_2, is primarily determined by the amount of hemoglobin in arterial blood that is saturated with oxygen.

$$CaO_2 = (Hgb \times 1.39 \times SaO_2) + (0.003 \times PaO_2)$$

REMEMBER: A quicker way to estimate this value: **Hgb × 1.39 × SaO₂**
Normal value: 15–24 volume percentage

ASSIST/CONTROL VENTILATION (see Ventilator Patterns)

ASTHMA

Asthma is from the Greek for "to pant." Hallmarks are tenacious sputum and reversible airway obstruction. Patient is dehydrated (related to tachypnea) and has decreased vesicular breath sounds with hyperexpansion of chest and decreased chest wall excursion. There is severe airway obstruction and respiratory acidosis. (In less severe attacks, there may be a decrease in the PCO_2 related to hyperventilation and respiratory alkalosis.)

- **Treatment of choice:** Aminophylline, steroids, hydration.

ATROPINE (see Respiratory Inhalation Medications)

BiPAP VENTILATOR SUPPORT

Bilevel positive airway pressure is a noncontinuous, noninvasive ventilation system used to augment breathing for patients who feel that CPAP is unbearable because it is too difficult to exhale against the back pressure. It is helpful for patients who have difficulty breathing (often at night) related to COPD, CHF, cystic fibrosis, sleep apnea syndrome, and neuromuscular diseases resulting in respiratory insufficiency. It does not provide total ventilator requirements and should never be used as a life-support device.

(continued)

NOTES

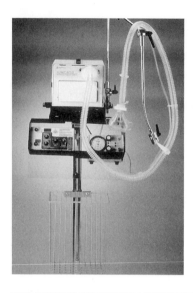

Figure 3-5 BiPAP machine for bilevel pressure therapy. (Courtesy of Respironics, Inc.)

◖ BLEB (see also Bulla)

A bleb is a small bulla, usually found in the subpleural zone of the lung abutting the pleura.

◖ BOYLE'S LAW

When the pressure of a gas is doubled and the temperature remains constant, the volume of the gas is reduced by one-half. At a constant temperature (T), the volume of a gas (V) is inversely proportional to the pressure (P) of the volume. That pressure remains constant if the temperature is unchanged.

$$P_1V_1 = P_2V_2$$

◖ BREATH SOUNDS, NORMAL

Bronchial breath sounds are normal over the upper third of the sternum and trachea. If they are heard anywhere else, they are abnormal. The sound is produced by the air movement through the larynx, setting up vibrations, **not** by the air leaving the alveoli. The sound is loud and high pitched.

Bronchovesicular breath sounds are heard over the lower two portions of the sternum, just to either side. They are heard posteriorly between the scapulae. If they are heard anywhere else, it is due to partial atelectasis or pulmonary consolidation. The sound is soft with a lower pitch.

(continued)

Vesicular breath sounds (inspiration) are produced by air entering the alveoli directly, separating the alveoli. They can be heard anywhere anteriorly, and posteriorly, they can be heard anywhere except between the scapulae. The sound is soft and breezy, with the lowest pitch.

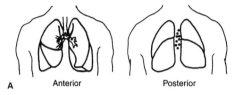

A   Anterior   Posterior

Bronchovesicular Breath Sounds

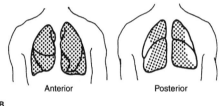

B   Anterior   Posterior

Vesicular Breath Sounds

FIGURE 3-6 The locations at which bronchovesicular breath sounds *(A)* and vesicular breath sounds *(B)* are normally auscultated. (Courtesy of Terry Des Jardins.)

⬤ BREATH SOUNDS, ABNORMAL

Rales (crackles) can be heard usually on inspiration only and are found wherever the underlying pathology is. The sound is similar to rubbing strands of hair together, next to the ear. They correlate with early left-sided failure, and the degree to which they are audible corresponds to the degree of the failure. They also may be caused by interstitial lung disease and pneumonias. If the rales disappear with three or four breaths or with a cough, they are not due to fluid, but to the actual separating of the alveolar walls. They are then known as dry rales, atelectatic rales, or hypostatic rales. Rales are common after 24 hours on bed rest.

Rhonchi are heard predominantly on expiration and are related to secretions in larger airways. The sound is of a continuous snoring quality, similar to rubbing two inflated balloons together.

Wheezes can be heard on inspiration or expiration. When breathing is partially constricted (as in asthma), the sound can be heard primarily on expiration. It has a musical quality, or is likened to creaking or groaning.

A **rub** is caused by the parietal and visceral pleura rubbing due to inflammation. The sound stops if the patient holds his breath. A rub is usually heard on inspiration **and** expiration and is a superficial squeaking or grating sound, similar to rubbing two pieces of leather together.

◯ BREATHING PATTERNS (see Respiratory Patterns)

◯ BRETHINE (see Respiratory Inhalation Medications)

◯ BRONCHITIS

The patient with bronchitis has recurrent, excessive bronchial mucus secretion resulting in a productive cough. The increased secretions often render the patient a perfect host for bacteria. The description of "blue bloater" is often given because of the presence of hypoxemia resulting in cyanosis and the tendency toward edema. Treatment is aimed at improving alveolar ventilation and relieving the hypoxemia through vigorous pulmonary toilet, postural drainage, IPPB therapy, bronchodilators, and mucolytic agents.

◯ BRONKOSOL (see Respiratory Inhalation Medications)

◯ BULLA

A thin-walled, localized pocket of air in lung tissue. Bullae vary in size from being barely visible on X-ray film to several centimeters in diameter. They may occur in otherwise normal lungs or may be a result of primary emphysema. Secondary infections often develop.

◯ CARBON MONOXIDE POISONING (see also Hyperbaric Oxygen, Oxyhemoglobin Dissociation Curve)

Carbon monoxide, with affinity for hemoglobin 210 times greater than oxygen, combines with hemoglobin (Hgb) to form carboxyhemoglobin (COHb). Carbon monoxide impairs oxygen unloading at the tissue level, and the oxyhemoglobin dissociation curve shifts to the left. This results in decreased O_2 available to tissues, creating cerebral hypoxia. The patient presents with a characteristic cherry red skin color and flulike symptoms, such as headache, nausea, vomiting, fatigue, and weakness. Treatment is with 100% oxygen until all signs and symptoms resolve. Hyperbaric oxygen therapy can be used to decrease the half-life, but due to the poor availability of HBO chambers, it's use is limited.

(continued)

NOTES

TABLE 3-3. Carboxyhemoglobin Levels

Carboxyhemoglobin Level	Symptoms
0–5%	Normal
<15%	Often in smokers, truck drivers
15–40%	Headache, some degree of confusion
40–60%	Loss of consciousness, Cheyne-Stokes respirations
50–70%	Mortality >50%

CHEST TUBES (see also Effusion, Pneumothorax)

Chest tubes are used in patients who require removal of air, blood, or fluid from the pleural or mediastinal space. Tube sizes are in French (F), the larger ones, 20F to 36F, being for blood and thick drainage, and the smaller ones, 16F to 20F, for removing air. Chest tube systems can be a one-, two-, or three-bottle setup or a disposable water-filled or dry system. The principle for all is the same: suction is applied (via submersion of the tube in a bottle system or connection to a suction source in the disposable system) usually to −20 cm H_2O. The water seal is a one-way valve that allows air to leave the pleural cavity but prevents it from returning, thereby maintaining a negative pressure. The collection chamber holds the drainage; >200 mL/hr indicates a bleeding complication.

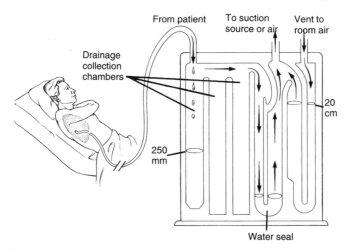

FIGURE 3-7 Disposable chest tube drainage system.

CHEST X-RAY FILM, NORMAL

When X-ray films are interpreted, the degrees of blackness on the film are compared either with each other or against a film taken earlier, providing a baseline. There are four types of densities (or blackness) seen on a chest film:

1. Gas or air: Least dense, absorbs minimal X rays, and appears *blackest.*

2. Water: Seen with soft tissue, muscle, blood. Heart appears as water density, which is lighter than gas density.

3. Fat.

4. Metal: *Lightest* of all densities, seen in bony structures such as ribs. Absorbs most X rays.

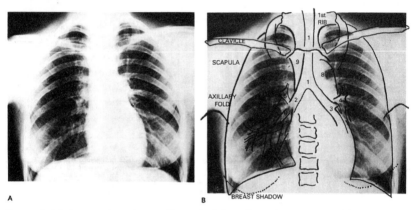

A   B

FIGURE 3-8 (A) Normal PA chest radiograph. **(B)** Outline of structures visible on normal PA chest radiograph. (Adapted from Fraser, R.G., Pare, J.A.P., et al. [1988]. *Diagnosis of disease of the chest* [pp. 288–290]. Philadelphia: WB Saunders. Reprinted with permission.)

CHEST X-RAY FILM, ABNORMAL

TABLE 3-4. Abnormal Chest X-Ray Appearances and Causes

Appearances	Possible Causes
Decreased volume: reduced size of thoracic cage, elevated diaphragms, increased interstitial markings	Decreased surfactant, decreased compliance, atelectasis
Increased volume: increased size of thoracic cage (increased hyperaeration), flattened diaphragm, reduced interstitial markings	Trapped air: emphysema, asthma, increased PEEP, increased mechanical ventilation volumes, pneumothorax (tension)

(continued)

TABLE 3-4. Abnormal Chest X-Ray Appearances and Causes (Continued)

Appearances	Possible Causes
Reticular pattern: irregular network of straight or curved densities	Interstitial infiltrates or fibrosis
Nodular pattern: confluent densities of different sizes	Increased interstitial or alveolar pattern
Ground glass	ARDS, certain infections
Air bronchogram: can visualize airways out towards the periphery	Any alveolar filling process, eg, pneumonia, edema
Miliary pattern: small, round regular densities	Interstitial micronodular pattern suggestive of disseminated granulomatous disease or metastatic malignancy
Decreased peripheral markings: decreased or absent markings in periphery	Air in pleural space, pulmonary hypertension, pulmonary embolism, emphysema
Costophrenic blunting: rounded angle	Fluid in pleural space
Increased heart size:	
Right ventricle: pulmonary artery pushed towards left cardiac border	Cor pulmonale
Right atrium	Cor pulmonale
Left ventricle: rounding of left cardiac border and boot-shaped extension	Congestive heart failure
Left atrium: lateral projection of right cardiac border	Congestive heart failure
Dilated pulmonary arteries: antler shaped, cloudiness at base	Pulmonary hypertension
Butterfly pattern:	
Puffy cloudiness in central lung fields	Pulmonary edema
Honeycomb cloudiness throughout lung fields	Interstitial edema
Kerley B lines: perpendicular lines to pleura in peripheral bases	Interstitial edema, dilated lymphatic vessels
AP projection vs PA projection: decreased volumes (unable to take deep breath), elevated hemidiaphragms, increased lung markings in bases, heart enlarged, scapula overlies upper fields, often rotated	Portable X-ray film, usually taken for bed-ridden patients (especially while on mechanical ventilation)
Silhouette sign: loss of the normal silhouette of the heart, aorta, or diaphragm	Water density (infiltrates) in anatomic contact with heart, aorta, or diaphragm

Adapted from Oaks, D. (1994) *Clinical Practitioners Guide to Respiratory Care.* Old Town, ME: Health Educator Publications. With permission.

CHRONIC OBSTRUCTIVE PULMONARY DISEASE

Chronic obstructive pulmonary disease (COPD) is a group of those respiratory diseases that obstruct the pathway of normal alveolar ventilation, either by spasm of the airways, mucus secretions, or morphopathologic changes of airways and/or alveoli. Three most common are (1) chronic bronchitis, (2) pulmonary emphysema, and (3) bronchial asthma.

Signs typically include elevated pulmonary artery pressures, peaked P on EKG tracing (pulmonary hypertension causes right atrial enlargement and position change), incomplete right bundle branch block, increased functional residual capacity (and barrel chest), multifocal atrial tachycardia (due to hypoxia and right ventricular strain), and compensatory polycythemia (increase in RBCs to increase the hematocrit).

Treatment is to first treat the hypoxia with vigorous pulmonary toilet and postural toilet, then give IPPB therapy (to aerate alveoli and remove CO_2), bronchodilator therapy, mucolytic agents, antibiotics (usually ampicillin), or steroids. Venturi mask delivers most controlled O_2 for patient.

CLOSED PNEUMOTHORAX (see Pneumothorax)

COMPLIANCE

Static compliance is a measurement of the elastic properties of the lung, usually measured while the patient is on the ventilator. A reduction in compliance also tends to reduce a patient's tidal volume and increase breathing frequency to overcome the work of moving large volumes of air. To calculate:

Tidal volume ÷ (plateau pressure minus PEEP)
Normal: (textbook) 100 mL/cm H_2O
(usually) 50 mL/cm H_2O

Dynamic compliance is a measurement to evaluate the work of breathing or the amount of force needed to overcome airway resistance. To calculate:

Tidal volume ÷ (peak inspiratory pressure minus PEEP)
Normal: 45 to 50 mL/cm H_2O

Studies have shown that as dead space to tidal volume ratios are increased, compliance falls, which is an indicator the patient's status is deteriorating.

CONTROLLED MECHANICAL VENTILATION (see Ventilator Patterns)

○ **COPD** (see Chronic Obstructive Pulmonary Disease)

○ **CPAP** (see Ventilator Patterns)

○ **CUFF MEASUREMENT** (see Endotracheal Tube Placement)

○ **DEAD SPACE**

Dead space is a measurement to determine total wasted ventilation or that which is ineffective in gas exchange. It is normally one-third of tidal volume, but this may increase markedly in the late phase of ARDS or in pulmonary embolism.

○ **DYNAMIC COMPLIANCE** (see Compliance)

○ **EFFUSION** (see also Pneumothorax)

Also known as hydrothorax, effusion is clinically the same as pneumothorax, but an effusion has fluid infiltrates instead of air. An empyema has puslike fluid. A pleural effusion shows blunting of the costophrenic angle on X-ray film, silhouetting of the diaphragm, and meniscus sign.

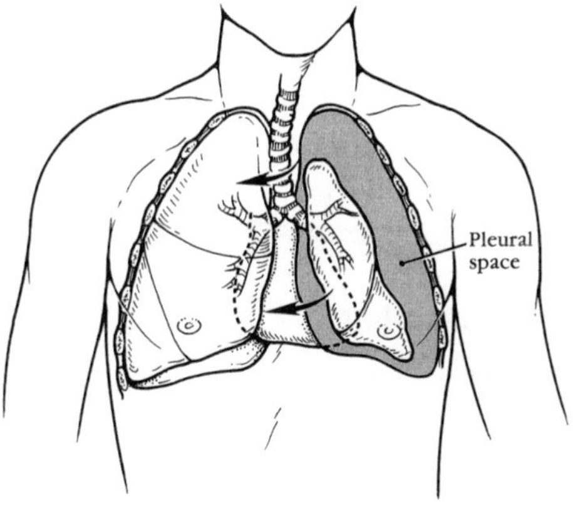

Pleural space

FIGURE 3-9 Pleural effusion. Fluid has collected in the pleural space and has displaced lung tissue. Also note the shift of fluid into the mediastinum and torsion of the bronchus.

○ **EMBOLISM** (see Pulmonary Embolism)

⬛ EMPHYSEMA (see also Chronic Obstructive Pulmonary Disease)

From the Greek for *inflation*, emphysema is an obstructive respiratory disorder characterized by air trapped in overdistended alveoli and collapse of bronchioles on expiration, causing prolongation of expiratory outflow. The lungs are hyperresonant with chest percussion. Even in the presence of severe disease, the patient maintains a normal gas exchange and often has an elevated hematocrit; thus, the term "pink puffer" is often applied.

⬛ EMPYEMA (see Effusion)

⬛ ENDOTRACHEAL TUBE PLACEMENT

Oral tube sizes:

Males 8.0 to 8.5 ID

Females 7.0 to 8.0 ID

Placement:

Should be 2 to 3 cm above the carina, where the trachea splits to main stem bronchi.

REMEMBER: **For a female:**

21 (cm) is lots of fun

22 (cm) will seldom do

23 (cm) should rarely be

Cuff pressures:

20 to 25 mmHg is usual

>25 mmHg = risk of tracheal damage

<20 mmHg = risk of aspiration around cuff

Optimum = enough air to barely seal trachea

⬛ EXTUBATION CRITERIA (see Weaning Parameters)

NOTES

◐ FICK PRINCIPLE (see also Swan-Ganz: Hemodynamic Normals in Part 2, Cardiovascular System)

Gas diffusion in the lung is described by Fick as "The total uptake or release of a substance by an organ is the product of the blood flow to the organ and of the arteriovenous concentrations of the substance."* This principle implies then, that the cardiac output per minute from the right ventricle (and consequently the left ventricle) can be determined by measuring the amount of blood the right ventricle pumps into the lung capillaries in one minute. Hence the formula:

$$\frac{O_2 \text{ absorption mL / min } (\dot{V}O_2)}{\underset{(CaO_2)}{\overset{O_2 \text{ content of}}{\text{arterial blood}}} \quad minus \quad \underset{(C\bar{v}O_2)}{\overset{O_2 \text{ content of}}{\text{mixed venous blood}}}} = \text{Cardiac output (CO)}$$

*Fick, 1870.

◐ FLAIL CHEST

Flail chest is a term used to describe an injury in which two or more ribs are fractured in several places, causing instability to the chest wall and subsequent respiratory impairment. Because the injured portion of the chest wall no longer has a bony connection with the rest of the rib cage, as the chest wall expands during inspiration, the detached part of the chest (flail segment) is drawn in and the mediastinum shifts away from the affected side. In expiration, the positive pressure pushes the flail segment outward, pulling the mediastinum toward the affected side and causing the patient difficulty exhaling. Usually, the injured ribs heal without intervention.

REMEMBER:

Inspiration: Chest wall moves **in.** Mediastinum moves **away** from affected side.

Expiration: Chest wall moves **out.** Mediastinum moves **toward** affected side.

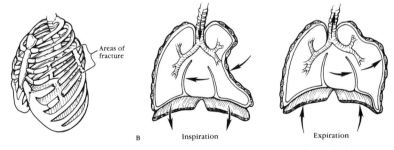

FIGURE 3-10 (A) Chest wall injury that can produce flail chest abnormality. **(B)** Physiology of flail chest abnormality resulting in paradoxical breathing.

◑ FORCED VITAL CAPACITY (see Weaning Parameters)

◑ FREMITUS

Fremitus is a vibration that can be palpated when a patient speaks. Sound is best produced through solid material, therefore:

Increased fremitus = lung consolidation, atelectasis

Decreased fremitus = pneumothorax, emphysema, effusions

REMEMBER: If you knock on a **solid** table, the sound is **greater** than if you knock on air.

◑ FUNCTIONAL RESIDUAL CAPACITY (see Lung Volumes)

◑ HEMOTHORAX (see Pneumothorax)

◑ HENDERSON-HASSELBALCH EQUATION

The Henderson-Hasselbalch equation is a method of calculating the pH of a buffer system. In medicine, it is used to calculate any one of the three parameters of acid-base balance: pH, $PaCO_2$, or bicarbonate.

$$pH = 6.1 + \log \frac{(HCO_3^- \text{ meq}/L)}{(0.03 \times PaCO_2)}$$

As long as the ratio of carbonic acid (H_2CO_3) to bicarbonate (HCO_3^-) is approximately 1:20, the pH of blood is normal. It is this ratio that determines the blood pH, rather than the absolute values of each.

(continued)

NOTES

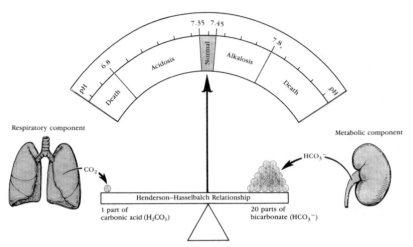

FIGURE 3-11 Henderson–Hasselbalch relationship demonstrating mechanisms for the defense against changes in body fluid pH.

⭕ HYDROTHORAX (see Effusion)

⭕ HYPERBARIC OXYGEN

Hyperbaric oxygen is found to be an effective agent against tissue infection such as chronic leg ulcers or gas gangrene. Unfortunately, after prolonged use, it induces endarteritis obliterans of small arterioles, defeating the benefits of the therapy. It is used occasionally in life-threatening cases of carbon monoxide poisoning by increasing the dissolved oxygen to maintain life while the carbon monoxide is displaced from hemoglobin.

⭕ HYPERCAPNIA

Hypercapnia is increased carbon dioxide in the blood resulting from hypoventilation due to respiratory muscle weakness, neurologic disease states, or drugs. With an increase in CO_2 production, the CO_2 diffuses rapidly into the blood. The pH falls, respirations increase, and respiratory acidosis results. Treatment is based on increasing alveolar ventilation.

⭕ HYPOCAPNIA

Hypocapnia is caused by hyperventilation due to pain, anxiety, liver disease, or CNS events. The increased alveolar ventilation results in a decreased CO_2 and an increase in pH. Treatment is to slow the respiratory rate and decrease the tidal volume, if high.

◑ HYPOXEMIA (see also Hypoxia)

Hypoxemia is a deficiency of O_2 tension in arterial blood, threatening tissue oxygenation. However, normal tissue oxygenation, even though hypoxemia is present, is possible through the compensatory mechanisms of (1) right shift of the oxyhemoglobin dissociation curve, (2) an increase in hemoglobin, or (3) an increase in cardiac output.

◑ HYPOXIA (see also Hypoxemia, Carbon Monoxide Poisoning)

Hypoxia is a deficiency of O_2 at the cellular level due to low cardiac output, arterial hypoxemia, or severe anemia. It results in anaerobic metabolism and lactic acidosis (regional or systemic). Treatment is to restore the O_2 deficiency with supplemental oxygen.

◑ INTERMITTENT MANDATORY VENTILATION (see Ventilator Patterns)

◑ INVERSE RATIO VENTILATION

The normal inspiratory/expiratory ventilation ratio in most ventilators is $1:1.5$ to $1:3$, producing a short inspiratory time and a long expiratory time. This increases venous return and right atrial filling, and allows time for air to leave the lungs.

Inverse ratio ventilation reverses this ratio to produce an inspiratory time equal to or even longer than expiratory time, as high as $4:1$. Although it is useful in ARDS (by expanding stiff alveoli slowly, and preventing their collapse with a rapid expiratory time), this mode is unnatural and requires the patient to be either heavily sedated, or more frequently, medically paralyzed.

(continued)

NOTES

TABLE 3-5. Inverse Ratio Ventilation

Inspiration Time (%)	Pause Time (%)	I : E Ratio
20	0	1 : 4
20	5	1 : 3
25	0	1 : 3
20	10	1 : 2.3
25	5	1 : 2.3
33	0	1 : 2
25	10	1 : 1.9
33	5	1 : 1.6
20	20	1 : 1.5
33	10	1 : 1.3
25	20	1 : 1.2
20	30	1 : 1
50	0	1 : 1
33	20	1.1 : 1
25	30	1.2 : 1
50	5	1.2 : 1
50	10	1.5 : 1
33	30	1.7 : 1
67	0	2 : 1
50	20	2.3 : 1
67	5	2.6 : 1
67	10	3.4 : 1
67	20*	4 : 1
80	0	4 : 1

*Reduced to 13%.

● **ISOETHARINE** (see Respiratory Inhalation Medications)

● **ISUPREL** (see Respiratory Inhalation Medications)

● **LUNG SOUNDS** (see Breath Sounds)

● **LUNG VOLUMES** (see also Weaning Parameters)

See Figure 3-12 on p. 148.

(*continued*)

ERV
Expiratory reserve volume
Maximum volume of air that can be exhaled after a normal exhalation to functional residual capacity. Usually $1/3$ of vital capacity.

IC
Inspiratory capacity
Volume of air exhaled after a normal exhalation. Usually $2/3$ of vital capacity.

ERV + IC
VC
Vital capacity
Maximum volume of air exhaled after a maximum inspiration. Useful to monitor this parameter in patients with neuromuscular disease or respiratory failure. Can be approximated at 65 cc/kg/body weight, but usually a graph is used to predict values. A decrease of VC in the neuromuscularly diseased patient indicates that the patient is unable to cough or move secretions (not true, however, if decrease is due to restrictive lung disease).

RV
Residual volume
Air that remains in lungs at the end of maximum exhalation

ERV + RV

FRC
Functional residual capacity
Volume of air in lungs after normal expiration.*

RV + VC
TLC
Total lung capacity
Volume of air in lungs after a maximal inspiration. The sum total of all lung volumes.

(V$_T$)
Tidal volume
As a component of VC, V_T is defined as the volume of air inspired and expired with each breath.

IRV
Inspiratory reserve volume
Maximum volume of air that can be inhaled after a tidal breath has been taken.

* Can be measured directly in a body plethysmograph, a wooden box shaped to fit the human frame in the sitting position, similar to a sauna bath. A transparent dome covers that part of the box where the head comes through. Once the patient is inside, the box is closed and becomes airtight. The plethysmograph incorporates the use of Boyle's Law (See Boyle's Law) to measure thoracic gas volume and has been found to yield much higher values for patients who have areas of the lung that do not communicate with the outside (e.g., where gas is trapped in emphysema or when a tumor occludes an airway.)

Figure 3-12 Lung volumes.

(continued)

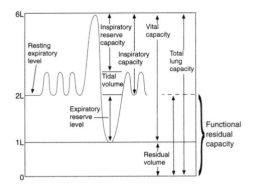

FIGURE 3-13 Pulmonary function test measurements showing normal lung volumes and capacity.

MECHANICAL VENTILATION (see Ventilator Patterns)

METAPROTERENOL SULFATE (see Respiratory Inhalation Medications)

MINUTE VENTILATION (see Weaning Parameters)

MIXED VENOUS ABGs (see also S$\bar{V}$O$_2$ Monitoring)

Mixed venous ABGs refers to a blood gas sample that indicates a complete mixing of the blood, that is, blood returned from the extremities to the right ventricle. This may sometimes be sampled from a central venous line, though even in the superior vena cava or right atrium, the mixing is incomplete. To be accurate, the sample must be obtained from the distal lumen of a pulmonary artery catheter.

pH	7.31–7.41
PCO$_2$ mmHg	41–51
PO$_2$ mmHg	35–42
O$_2$ saturation %	68–77
HCO$_3^-$ meq/L	22–26

FIGURE 3-14 Mixed venous ABG values.

NOTES

⬤ OBSTRUCTIVE DISEASES (see Chronic Obstructive Pulmonary Disease)

⬤ OPEN PNEUMOTHORAX (see Pneumothorax)

⬤ OXYGEN CONSUMPTION

Oxygen consumption calculation is used to determine the volume of oxygen consumed by the body tissues per minute, as indicated by the amount of oxygen delivered less the amount of oxygen returned after circulation.

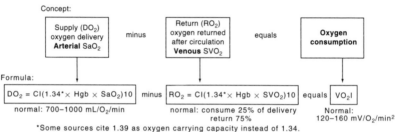

Concept:

| Supply (DO_2) oxygen delivery **Arterial** SaO_2 | minus | Return (RO_2) oxygen returned after circulation **Venous** SVO_2 | equals | **Oxygen consumption** |

Formula:

$DO_2 = CI(1.34^* \times Hgb \times SaO_2)10$ minus $RO_2 = CI(1.34^* \times Hgb \times SVO_2)10$ equals VO_2I

normal: 700–1000 mL/O_2/min   normal: consume 25% of delivery   Normal:
                                                  return 75%   120–160 mV/O_2/min[2]

*Some sources cite 1.39 as oxygen carrying capacity instead of 1.34.

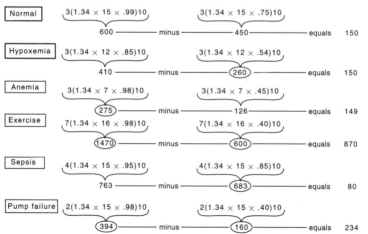

Transport pattern examples:

| Normal | $3(1.34 \times 15 \times .99)10$ | | $3(1.34 \times 15 \times .75)10$ | | |
| | 600 —— minus —— 450 —— equals | | | | 150 |

| Hypoxemia | $3(1.34 \times 12 \times .85)10$ | | $3(1.34 \times 12 \times .54)10$ | | |
| | 410 —— minus —— ⃝260 —— equals | | | | 150 |

| Anemia | $3(1.34 \times 7 \times .98)10$ | | $3(1.34 \times 7 \times .45)10$ | | |
| | ⃝275 —— minus —— 126 —— equals | | | | 149 |

| Exercise | $7(1.34 \times 16 \times .98)10$ | | $7(1.34 \times 16 \times .40)10$ | | |
| | ⃝1470 —— minus —— ⃝600 —— equals | | | | 870 |

| Sepsis | $4(1.34 \times 15 \times .95)10$ | | $4(1.34 \times 15 \times .85)10$ | | |
| | 763 —— minus —— ⃝683 —— equals | | | | 80 |

| Pump failure | $2(1.34 \times 15 \times .98)10$ | | $2(1.34 \times 15 \times .40)10$ | | |
| | ⃝394 —— minus —— ⃝160 —— equals | | | | 234 |

FIGURE 3-15 Oxygen consumption. *Circled numbers* indicate parameter out of balance.

⬤ OXYGEN DELIVERY SYSTEMS AND CONVERSIONS

TABLE 3-6. Oxygen Delivery Systems and Conversions

LOW FLOW FiO$_2$/Lpm (GROSS ESTIMATES)

NASAL CATHETER OR CANNULA

1 Lpm	24%
2 Lpm	28%
3 Lpm	32%
4 Lpm	36%
5 Lpm	40%
6 Lpm	44%

MASK (SIMPLE)

5–6 Lpm	40%
6–7 Lpm	50%
7–8 Lpm	60%

PARTIAL REBREATHER

6 Lpm	35%
8 Lpm	50%
10 Lpm	60%

NONREBREATHER

6 Lpm	60%
8 Lpm	80%

Lpm, liters per minute.

⬤ OXYGEN TOXICITY

Oxygen toxicity is best thought of as the truly poisonous effect of the drug oxygen on the whole body. It develops after breathing 100% O$_2$ for greater than 12 hours; it can occur with an FiO$_2$ below 100%, but for a greater length of time. An FiO$_2$ of less than 60% is probably safe for weeks. To avoid toxicity, however, the PaO$_2$ should be maintained at the lowest concentration possible, and the use of PEEP should be considered. Transfuse RBCs to anemics.

Symptoms of oxygen toxicity include dyspnea, decreased compliance, an increase in the A-a gradient, and parethesis in the extremities. Retrosternal pain is noted in some patients after as little as 6 hours on 100% oxygen. Complications from oxygen toxicity are on the decline with the sophisticated ventilation systems of today, although occasionally edema and ARDS may result.

(continued)

The concept of oxygen toxicity:

High % O_2
▽
Airways contain less nitrogen
▽
Nitrogen washout
▽
Alveoli contain only O_2, CO_2, and H_2O vapor
▽
Secretions occlude airway
▽
O_2 diffuses into capillary
▽
Nothing left in alveoli
▽
Alveolus collapses

 OXYHEMOGLOBIN DISSOCIATION CURVE

The oxyhemoglobin dissociation curve, a graph of great physiologic importance, demonstrates the relationship between PO_2 and O_2 saturation. The shape of the curve represents the protective mechanisms in health and disease. When there are large changes in the arterial PO_2 (upper portion of the graph), there are only small changes in the oxygen saturation. The lower, steeper portion of the curve shows that as hemoglobin becomes desaturated from 70% downward, large amounts of O_2 are released for utilization by tissues with proportionally less change in PO_2. Thus, the significance of the curve shows that:

1. A shift to the *left* means the RBCs hold on to oxygen (difficult to unload), less O_2 is delivered to the tissues, and therefore, *the O_2 saturation increases.*
Causes: alkalosis, hypothermia, decreased $PaCO_2$, or a drop in 2,3-DPG.

REMEMBER: **Left = aLkaLosis and coLd.**

2. A shift to the right means the RBCs readily release oxygen (better unloading at tissue level), and therefore the O_2 saturation readings decrease (*tissues* are OK, even though PO_2 and SaO_2 are low).
Causes: Acidosis, fever, increased $PaCO_2$, and a rise in 2,3-DPG.

REMEMBER: A shift to the **right** is **right** for the patient. (The O_2 saturation may be down, but there is less bound oxygen to the RBCs and more oxygen available to the tissues.)

(continued)

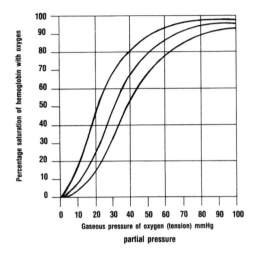

Gaseous pressure of oxygen (tension) mmHg

partial pressure

FIGURE 3-16 Right and left shifts of oxyhemoglobin dissociation curve.

PEEP (see Ventilator Patterns)

PNEUMONIA

Pathophysiology:

Inflammation (infection) of alveoli leading to consolidation
▽
Alveoli fill with exudate
▽
$\dot{V}/\dot{Q}$ mismatch
▽
Shunt

Frequently, pleural effusions develop (see Effusion). Best positioning for oxygenation is with good lung **down.**

NOTES

⬤ PNEUMOTHORAX

A pneumothorax is the collection of air in pleural space that disrupts negative pressure. There are several forms.

An **open pneumothorax** ("sucking chest wound") occurs when the outer chest wall is damaged and allows air to enter the lung. If the size of the hole in the chest wall is significantly smaller than the trachea, the patient can usually tolerate it for a short time. The air moving in and out contributes nothing to gas exchange, however, and inhibits lung expansion and increases work of breathing.

Treatment includes placement of chest tubes and an occlusive chest wall dressing.

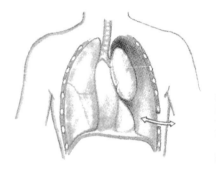

FIGURE 3-17 Open pneumothorax. (Hood, R.M. [1989]. Pre-hospital management, initial evaluation, and resuscitation. In R.M. Hood, A.D. Boyd, & A.T. Culliford [eds.], *Thoracic trauma* [p. 14]. Philadelphia: WB Saunders. Reprinted with permission.)

A **closed pneumothorax** (spontaneous) occurs when the outer chest wall is intact but damaged visceral pleura allow air to enter with no place to exit. It is usually caused by the rupture of a small bleb (an enlarged air sac) on the surface of the lung, overdistension of alveoli, or rupture of diseased lung. If the initial leak is small and no more air enters, the pneumothorax resolves spontaneously in a few days. If, however, the leak continues, more air enters, the pressure builds, and a tension pneumothorax results.

A **tension pneumothorax** occurs when air can't be evacuated from the pleura and the mediastinum is forced to the opposite side, sometimes causing collapse of the opposite lung as well. There is a decreased cardiac output and a decreased venous return. A tension pneumothorax is often related to PEEP, usually >15 (if the tidal volume used is too large).

(continued)

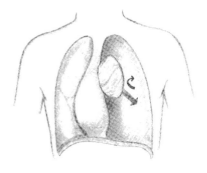

FIGURE 3-18 Tension pneumothorax. (Hood, R.M. [1989]. Pre-hospital management, initial evaluation, and resuscitation. In R.M. Hood, A.D. Boyd, & A.T. Culliford [eds.], *Thoracic trauma* [p. 14]. Philadelphia: WB Saunders. Reprinted with permission.)

A **hemothorax** is the same as a pneumothorax, but there is a collection of blood instead of air.

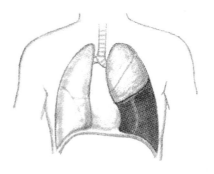

FIGURE 3-19 Massive hemothorax. (Hood, R.M. [1989]. Pre-hospital management, initial evaluation, and resuscitation. In R.M. Hood, A.D. Boyd, & A.T. Culliford [eds.], *Thoracic trauma* [p. 14]. Philadelphia: WB Saunders. Reprinted with permission.)

NOTES

● POSTURAL DRAINAGE POSITIONS

To drain the posterior lower lobes, position patient's head down 18° to 25° (hips elevated) with patient prone. Percuss lower ribs on both sides of spine.

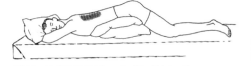

FIGURE 3-20 To drain the posterior lower lobes.

To drain the right lateral or left lateral lower lung segments, position patient on opposite side of lobe to be drained (ie, to drain right lobe, patient lies on left side), with head down 15° (hips elevated). Percuss lower ribs beneath axilla.

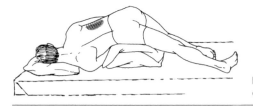

FIGURE 3-21 To drain the right lateral lower lung segments.

To drain the anterior lower lung segments, position patient on back with hips elevated 16 to 18 inches with pillows.

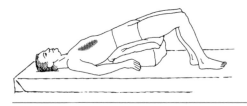

FIGURE 3-22 To drain the anterior lower lung segments.

To drain the upper lung fields, raise head of bed up 30° to 45°, with patient in a semireclining position.

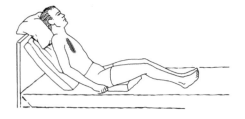

FIGURE 3-23 To drain the upper lung field and allow more forceful coughing.

(*continued*)

To drain the right or left lower lobes, patient lies on opposite side of lobe to be drained (ie, to drain the left, patient lies on the right). Patient's hips should be elevated on pillows to form a 30° to 45° angle. Percuss lower ribs.

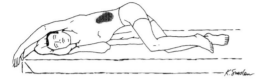

FIGURE 3-24 To drain the left lower lobes.

⬤ **PRESSURE CONTROL** (see Ventilator Patterns)

⬤ **PRESSURE SUPPORT** (see Ventilator Patterns)

⬤ **PROVENTIL** (see Respiratory Inhalation Medications)

⬤ **PULMONARY EDEMA**

Pulmonary edema is the accumulation of fluid in the interstitial spaces of the lung or in the air spaces themselves, causing impaired gas exchange. High pressure pulmonary edema (cardiogenic, hydrostatic) is related to volume/pressure overload of pulmonary system. Transudation of fluid into the alveoli occurs, causing an elevation of colloid osmotic pressure. This, in turn, results in fluid being forced into the alveoli. One cause of the increased capillary pressure is the dam effect from the left ventricle back through the pulmonary circulation present in left ventricular failure and pericardial disease. The cornerstone of treatment is 100% O_2, furosemide (Lasix), and morphine.

Low pressure pulmonary edema (noncardiogenic, neurogenic) is related to the increased permeability of the pulmonary capillary membrane due to ARDS, increased ICP, hemorrhage, trauma, or stroke. The treatment centers around supportive care rather than morphine or Lasix.

Both types of edema are characterized by dyspnea; cough; orthopnea; anxiety; cyanosis; sweating; pink frothy sputum; and, very often, chest pressure.

(continued)

NOTES

Pathophysiology of pulmonary edema (oversimplified):

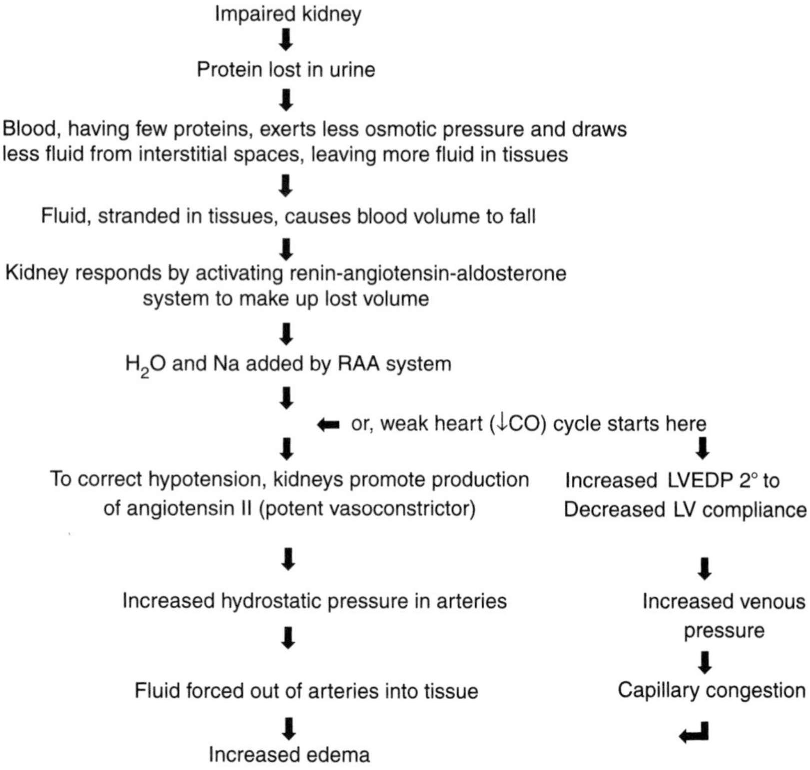

Impaired kidney
↓
Protein lost in urine
↓
Blood, having few proteins, exerts less osmotic pressure and draws
less fluid from interstitial spaces, leaving more fluid in tissues
↓
Fluid, stranded in tissues, causes blood volume to fall
↓
Kidney responds by activating renin-angiotensin-aldosterone
system to make up lost volume
↓
H_2O and Na added by RAA system
↓
← or, weak heart (↓CO) cycle starts here
↓   ↓
To correct hypotension, kidneys promote production   Increased LVEDP 2° to
of angiotensin II (potent vasoconstrictor)   Decreased LV compliance
↓   ↓
Increased hydrostatic pressure in arteries   Increased venous
↓   pressure
↓
Fluid forced out of arteries into tissue   Capillary congestion
↓   ↵
Increased edema

FIGURE 3-25 An oversimplified flow chart depicting pulmonary edema.

⬤ PULMONARY EMBOLISM (see also V̇/Q̇ Ratio)

Pulmonary embolism is a sudden mechanical obstruction of at least 50% of the pulmonary arterial bed. It is related to ventilation/perfusion imbalance and shunting. About 90% of pulmonary emboli are due to deep vein thrombosis (iliac, femoral, vena cava). ABGs show decreased O_2 and decreased PCO_2 with respiratory alkalosis. The patient exhibits dyspnea, tachypnea, and chest pain, varying in degree from mild to severe. A pulmonary embolus may invert or depress the ST segment on the EKG and cause right axis deviation, atrial fibrillation, or right bundle branch block. Treatment is based on anticoagulating the patient with heparin and keeping the PTT 1.5 to 2 times normal. Streptokinase, urokinase, filters, and sometimes embolectomy are also used.

⬤ **PULMONARY VASCULAR RESISTANCE (see also Swan-Ganz: Hemodynamic Normals in Part 2, Cardiovascular System)**

The force the right ventricle needs to produce blood flow through the pulmonary system is the pulmonary vascular resistance (PVR). Normal is 37 to 250 dyne/sec/cm. Pulmonary vessels constrict with a fall in alveolar PO_2 or a rise in arterial PCO_2. Also, an obstruction (such as a pulmonary embolus) causes the PVR to rise.

⬤ **RACEMIC EPINEPHRINE (see Respiratory Inhalation Medications)**

⬤ **RENIN ANGIOTENSIN SYSTEM (see Renin Angiotensin System in Part 5, Renal System)**

⬤ **RESPIRATORY FAILURE (see Acute Respiratory Failure)**

⬤ **RESPIRATORY INHALATION MEDICATIONS**

Albuterol (Proventil, Ventolin)

Albuterol is a bronchodilator with minor β_1 and strong β_2 adrenergic receptor effects. Usual dose, by aerosol: 0.5 cc of 0.5% solution in 3 cc NS; by inhaler: 2 puffs tid or qid. Onset is in about 15 minutes, the peak 30 to 60 minutes, and the duration ranges from 3 to 8 hours. It is useful in patients with asthma or COPD. It can cause tachycardia, palpitations, insomnia. There is no advantage to administering albuterol for broncho-constriction.

Alupent (see Metaproterenol Sulfate)

Atropine

Atropine has an anticholinergic action to block acetylcholine and is useful for drying secretions. Onset is 15 minutes, peak ½ to 1 hour, and duration 3 to 4 hours. Usual dose, by aerosol: 0.05 to 0.1 mg/kg of a 1% solution. It can cause pupil dilation, increased CNS stimulation, tachycardia.

Brethine (Terbutaline)

Brethine is a long-acting bronchodilator. It stimulates some β_1 adrenergic receptors, but mostly β_2. Onset is 5 to 30 minutes, peak 30 to 60 minutes, and duration 3 to 6 hours. Usual dose, by aerosol: 0.25 to 0.5 cc in 2.5 cc NS every 4 to 8 hours; by inhaler: 2 puffs every 4 to 6 hours. It can cause

(continued)

vasodilation with a decrease in the blood pressure and an increase in the heart rate.

Bronkosol (see Isoetharine)

Isoetharine (Bronkosol)

Isoetharine has some β_1 and moderate β_2 properties. Onset is 1 to 5 minutes, peak 5 to 60 minutes, and duration 1 to 3 hours. Usual dose, by aerosol: 0.5 cc in 2.5 cc NS qid; by inhaler: 1 to 2 puffs qid. This is a good choice for patients with cardiac arrhythmias.

Isuprel (Isoproterenol)

Isuprel is a potent bronchodilator with strong β_1 and β_2 properties. It relaxes the smooth muscles of the bronchial tree and is a good drug choice for acute bronchospasm. Onset is 2 to 5 minutes, peak 5 to 60 minutes, and duration ½ to 3 hours. Usual dose by aerosol: 0.25 to 0.5 cc of a 5% solution in 2.5 cc NS qid; by inhaler: 1 to 2 puffs qid. Frequent side effects occur, including palpitations, tachycardia, and flushing of skin.

Metaproterenol Sulfate (Alupent)

Metaproterenol sulfate is a long-lasting bronchodilator that stimulates both β_1 and β_2 adrenergic receptors. The onset is 1 to 5 minutes, peak ½ to 1 hour, and duration 2 to 6 hours. Usual dose, by aerosol: 0.3 cc of a 5% solution in 2.5 cc NS qid; by inhaler: 2 to 3 puffs every 4 hours. It can cause tachycardia.

Mucomyst (Acetylcysteine)

Mucomyst is a mucolytic agent indicated for tenacious secretions. Liquefication is apparent within 1 minute following administration, with a maximum effect noted in 5 to 10 minutes. Usual dose, by aerosol: 3 to 5 cc of 20% Mucomyst in 5 cc solution given tid or qid; by instillation: 1 to 2 cc of 20% Mucomyst, or 2 to 4 cc of 10% Mucomyst.

Proventil (see Albuterol)

Racemic Epinephrine

Racemic epinephrine is a strong β_1 bronchodilator, useful for laryngospasm and immediate postextubation in children. Onset is 3 to 5 minutes, peak 5 to 20 minutes, with a duration of 1 to 3 hours. Usual dose, by aerosol: 0.125 to 0.5 cc in 2.5 cc NS; by inhaler: 1 to 2 puffs qid.

Ventolin (see Albuterol)

RESPIRATORY PATTERNS

Apneustic Breathing

Apneustic breathing is characterized by a prolonged inspiratory hold. There may be expiratory pauses. Typically, it has a very slow rate. It is related to midbrain or low pons problems.

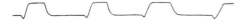

FIGURE 3-26 Apneustic breathing.

Ataxic (see Biot's Respirations)

Biot's Respirations

Biot's respirations are irregular and random with no pattern. Several short breaths of equal depths are followed by long, irregular periods of apnea. They are related to lesions at the midbrain or medullary level.

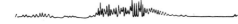

FIGURE 3-27 Ataxic breathing (Biot's respirations).

Central Neurogenic Hyperventilation

Central neurogenic hyperventilation looks like the hiccups. There are sustained, regular, rapid respirations with forced inspiration and expiration at a rate of >60 per minute. It is related to lesions in low midbrain or pons.

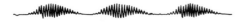

FIGURE 3-28 Central neurogenic hyperventilation.

Cheyne-Stokes Respirations

Cheyne-Stokes respirations are characterized by initial shallow respirations that increase in depth, reach a peak, then decline. A period of apnea follows, and the cycle is repeated. The apnea gives the PCO_2 time to build up again (after being blown off by the rapid respirations) and triggers the breathing pattern to start again. Cheyne-Stokes respirations occur with upper brain stem involvement.

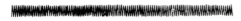

FIGURE 3-29 Cheyne-Stokes respirations.

Cluster Breathing

Cluster breathing denotes a lesion in the low pons. Periods of irregular respirations alternate with periods of apnea.

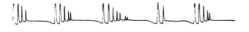

FIGURE 3-30 Cluster breathing.

(*continued*)

Kussmaul's Respirations

Kussmaul's respirations are characterized by deep, regular, sighing respirations, with an increase in respiratory rate. They are due to metabolic acidosis.

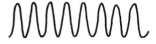

FIGURE 3-31 Kussmaul's respirations

 RESPIRATORY SYSTEM ANATOMY (see Anatomy, Pulmonary)

 RESPIRATORY PHYSIOLOGY TERMS AND SYMBOLS

TABLE 3-7. Respiratory Terms and Symbols

EXAMPLES*

PaO_2	partial pressure of oxygen in arterial blood
$PaCO_2$	partial pressure of carbon dioxide in arterial blood
PAO_2	partial pressure of oxygen in inspired gas
P_B	barometric pressure
V_T	tidal volume
V_D	volume of dead space
$\dot{V}_E$	volume of expired gas per unit of time (minute ventilation)
$\dot{V}_A$	volume of alveolar gas per unit of time (alveolar ventilation)

LUNG VOLUMES

VC	vital capacity	VT	tidal volume
IC	inspiratory capacity	TLC	total lung capacity
IRV	inspiratory reserve volume	EEP	end expiratory pressure
ERV	expiratory reserve volume	EPAP	end positive airway pressure
FRC	functional residual capacity	PIP	peak inspiratory pressure
RV	residual volume		

PULMONARY MECHANICS

MEFR	maximal expiratory flow rate	IE	inspiratory/expiratory ratio
MMFR	maximal mid-flow rate	FEF	forced expiratory flow rate
MIFR	maximal inspiratory flow rate	FVC	forced vital capacity
MVV	maximal voluntary ventilation	ECMO	extracorporeal membrane oxygenation
FEV	forced expiratory volume		
CV	closing volume	NIF	negative inspiratory force
CC	closing capacity	IRV	inverse ratio ventilation
FVC	forced vital capacity		

GENERAL

V	gas volume
$\dot{V}$	gas volume per unit of time
P	gas pressure in general
Q	volume of blood
$\dot{Q}$	volume flow of blood per unit of time
S	percent saturation of hemoglobin with oxygen or carbon monoxide
f	breathing frequency

(continued)

TABLE 3-7. Respiratory Terms and Symbols (Continued)

SECONDARY SYMBOLS

GAS PHASE ONLY

I	inspired gas
E	expired gas
D	dead space gas
A	alveolar gas
T	tidal gas
L	lung
B	barometric

BLOOD PHASE ONLY

a	arterial
v	venous
c	capillary

A dash above any symbol indicates a mean value.
*A dot above any symbol indicates a rate or time derivation.

RESTRICTIVE DISEASES

Restrictive diseases are those respiratory diseases that restrict movement of the thorax and/or lungs, resulting in decreased chest expansion and therefore a reduction in volume of air inspired and expired. They may be associated with interstitial fibrosis; thoracic deformities; or neurologic factors, such as, myasthenia gravis or Guillain-Barré.

REVERSE I : E RATIO (see Inverse Ratio Ventilation)

SPONTANEOUS PNEUMOTHORAX (see Pneumothorax)

STATIC COMPLIANCE (see Compliance)

S$\bar{V}$O$_2$ MONITORING: NORMALS (see also S$\bar{V}$O$_2$ Monitoring in Part 2, Cardiovascular System; Oxygen Consumption)

Mixed venous oxygen saturation reflects the body's ability to provide adequate O$_2$ in response to tissue oxygen demands. It is affected by (1) cardiac output, (2) hemoglobin, (3) arterial oxygen saturation, and (4) tissue oxygen consumption.

REMEMBER: When calibrating the S$\bar{V}$O$_2$ monitor draw waste, then sample from the distal part. Compare the monitored S$\bar{V}$O$_2$ value with the mixed venous O$_2$ saturation value, not the PO$_2$.

(*continued*)

Normal $S\overline{V}O_2$ = 60% to 77%
Normal mixed venous PO_2 = 25 to 40 mmHg
>77% = sepsis, left to right shunt, excess inotrope, hypothermia, cell poisoning, or wedged catheter
<60%* = cardiac decompensation
<50%* = lactic acidosis
<20%* = permanent damage
       *Sustained values

◻ **SYNCHRONIZED INTERMITTENT MANDATORY VENTILATION (see Ventilator Patterns)**

◻ **TENSION PNEUMOTHORAX (see Pneumothorax)**

◻ **TIDAL VOLUME (see Lung Volumes)**

◻ **TRACHEOSTOMY**

Shiley disposable cannula tubes are low-pressure, cuffed tracheostomy tubes, which are marked "DCT" on the swivel neck plate for easy reference while the tube is in situ. The initials ID indicate inner diameter, and the initials OD indicate outer diameter of the cannula. Length is the distance from the neck plate to the distal tip of the tube.

TABLE 3-8. Tracheostomy Tube Diameters and Conversion

Outside diameter (mm)	French	Jackson	Approximate inside diameter (mm)
4.3	13	00	2.5
5.0	15	0	3.0
5.5	16.5	1	3.5
6.0	18	2	4.0
7.0	21	3	4.5–5.0
8.0	24	4	5.5
9.0	27	5	6.0–6.5
10.0	30	6	7.0
11.0	33	7	7.5–8.0
12.0	36	8	8.5
13.0	39	9	9.0–9.5
14.0	42	10	10.0
15.0	45	11	10.5–11.0
16.0	48	12	11.5

(continued)

Fenestrated cuffs allow the patient to speak, but when capping a fenestrated cuffed tube, be sure to deflate the cuff and remove the inner cannula. This allows air to pass by the larynx instead of the stoma.

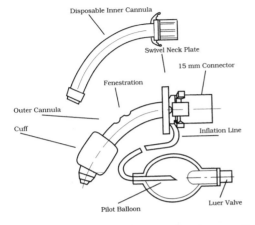

FIGURE 3-32 Shiley tracheostomy tube. (Courtesy of Mallinckrodt Medical, Irvine, CA)

NOTES

V̇/Q̇ Ratio

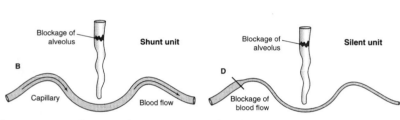

FIGURE 3-33 Ventilation-perfusion situations: **(A)** Normal ventilation, normal perfusion; **(B)** shunting with no ventilation, normal perfusion; **(C)** dead space with normal ventilation, no perfusion; **(D)** silent with no ventilation, no perfusion.

Optimum gas exchange between blood and the alveolus occurs when ventilation and perfusion correspond equally. Normally, a ratio of 4 L/min ventilation : 5 L/min perfusion occurs in a healthy individual, yielding a V̇/Q̇ ratio 0.8 : 1. A mismatch is said to exist when there is inadequate ventilation, perfusion, or both. Anything that interferes with ventilation (bronchospasm, emphysema, asthma, and so forth) will decrease the V̇/Q̇ ratio, and anything that interferes with perfusion (pulmonary embolus, changes in pulmonary artery pressures, and so forth) will increase the V̇/Q̇ ratio.

VENOUS O$_2$ CONTENT

Venous oxygen content, or $C\overline{v}O_2$, is primarily determined by the amount of hemoglobin in venous blood that is saturated with oxygen.

$$C\overline{v}O_2 = (Hgb \times 1.39 \times S\overline{v}O_2) + 1.39 \times S\overline{v}O_2$$

REMEMBER **this faster calculation for a quick approximation:**

$$C\overline{v}O_2 = (Hgb \times 1.39 \times S\overline{v}O_2)$$

Normal value: 12–15 volume percent

⬤ VENTILATION/PERFUSION RATIO (see V̇/Q̇ Ratio)

⬤ VENTILATOR PATTERNS

Assist/Control Mode

Assist/control (AC) mode allows the frequency of breaths and tidal volume to be preset by the ventilator, but the patient has the option of initiating inspiration as desired. However, *the preset tidal volume must always be given.* There is a backup rate, but the patient may overbreathe this rate.

Controlled Mechanical Ventilation

Controlled mechanical ventilation (CMV) is basically the same as assist/control mode, but the frequency of breaths is determined by the ventilator alone, with no option available to the patient. In patients with neurologic events, those with sedation on board, or paralyzed patients, it is sometimes necessary to render the ventilator insensitive to the patient's inspiratory efforts to achieve controlled ventilation.

Continuous Positive Airway Pressure

Continuous positive airway pressure (CPAP) is pressure that is maintained throughout inspiration and expiration during spontaneous breathing. It is usually 5 to 15 cm H_2O. Patient may generate own rate of breathing and own tidal volume, thus, CPAP may be used alone or with IMV at low rates for weaning.

Flow-by Ventilation

Flow-by ventilation, like pressure support, produces a continuous flow of gas through the circuit, which can meet the patient's demands but not assist the patient's ventilation. However, because the ventilator circuit is not closed (as in pressure support), flow-by ventilation cannot ventilate like high pressure support levels can. The fact that it is not pressurized, however, is an advantage in that there is no risk of barotrauma. It is often used as a weaning mode in conjunction with assist/control or pressure support. (It converts the system from pressure to flow triggered.)

Intermittent Mandatory Ventilation

Intermittent mandatory ventilation (IMV) requires the ventilator to deliver a predetermined number of breaths and set tidal volume. It allows the patient to breathe spontaneously between machine breaths, but the patient receives only his own spontaneous tidal volume. IMV can be used as a method of weaning.

(continued)

Positive End-Expiratory Pressure

Positive end-expiratory pressure (PEEP) is positive pressure, usually 5 to 20 cm H_2O, added at the end of expiration. It prevents the closure of the alveoli and promotes better oxygen exchange. It is used as an adjunct to assist/control, intermittent mandatory ventilation, synchronized intermittent mandatory ventilation, and pressure support modes. High levels of PEEP may cause barotrauma to weak lungs and may result in a tension pneumothorax, or they may decrease cardiac output by increasing intrathoracic pressure, causing compression of the heart and decreased venous return. The patient usually responds to volume to maintain adequate preload.

REMEMBER: **PEEP is DEEP** (cardiac output is down).

Pressure Control

Pressure control (PC) is a setting by which pressure and respiratory rate are predetermined. The ventilator delivers a flow of gas until the preset pressure is attained. It can be used with inverse ratio ventilation to allow alveoli a prolonged duration of positive inflation. This, in turn, shortens expiratory time and prevents loss of the patient's tidal volume.

Pressure Support

Pressure support (PS) is a weaning method whereby the patient initiates inspiration and the ventilator supports (assists) to achieve a predetermined peak pressure level. This eases the flow of gas into the lungs and increases tidal volume.

Synchronized Intermittent Mandatory Ventilation

Synchronized intermittent mandatory ventilation (SIMV) is essentially the same as IMV, but the ventilator is synchronized so that if a patient initiates a breath, the ventilator does not deliver a breath at the same time. It is a method of weaning that is more comfortable for the patient than IMV.

VENTOLIN (see Respiratory Inhalation Medications)

VITAL CAPACITY (see Lung Volumes)

WEANING PARAMETERS (see also Lung Volumes)

All criteria need not be satisfied:

Forced vital capacity (FVC) (maximum exhalation after maximum inhalation): **10 to 15 mL/kg.**

Tidal volume (VT): **5 mL/kg.**

Negative inspiratory force (NIF) (indicates how much negative pressure can be generated): if not **at least −20 cm,** patient cannot usually maintain minute volume. Normal: −80 cm to −100 cm.

$PaO_2 > 80\%.$

Respiratory rate: **>12 and <30** breaths/min.

Minute volume (MV) (amount of air in and out in one minute). **Normal: 5 to 10 L/min.**

<5 L/min indicates patient probably won't wean.

Weaning may be unsuccessful if:

Heart rate is elevated or decreased by 20 beats per minute from baseline.

Heart rate is below 60.

Blood pressure is elevated or decreased by 20 mmHg from baseline.

Respiratory rate is <8 or >25 breaths per minute.

Pulmonary capillary wedge pressure is greater than 20 mmHg.

Negative inspiratory force (NIF) is below −20 cm.

Minute volume (MV) is <5 L/min.

The frequency/tidal volume (f/VT) ratio is >105. (Twenty percent of patients <105 may still fail.) To calculate f/VT, divide respiratory rate by tidal volume.

X-RAY FILM (see Chest X-Ray Film)

PART
4

Gastrointestinal and Urinary Systems

ANATOMY, DIGESTIVE SYSTEM

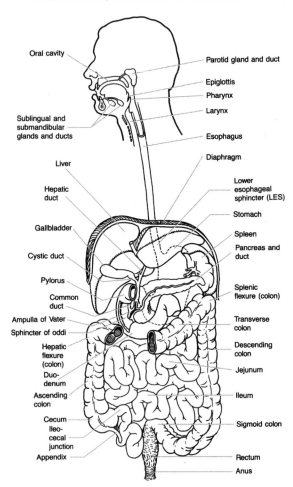

Oral cavity

Parotid gland and duct

Epiglottis
Pharynx
Larynx

Sublingual and
submandibular
glands and ducts

Esophagus

Liver

Diaphragm

Hepatic
duct

Lower
esophageal
sphincter (LES)

Stomach

Gallbladder

Spleen

Pancreas and
duct

Cystic duct

Pylorus

Splenic
flexure (colon)

Common
duct

Transverse
colon

Ampulla of Vater

Sphincter of oddi

Descending
colon

Hepatic
flexure
(colon)

Duo-
denum

Jejunum

Ascending
colon

Ileum

Cecum
Ileo-
cecal
junction

Sigmoid colon

Appendix

Rectum

Anus

FIGURE 4-1 The diges-
tive tract.

ANATOMY: LIVER FUNCTION (see also Bilirubin)

The liver is the largest internal organ. It stores fat-soluble vitamins and conjugates bilirubin to make it water soluble for excretion by the kidneys. In hepatic failure, the liver is unable to conjugate bilirubin, leading to an increase in both direct and indirect bilirubin, as well as a buildup of ammonia.

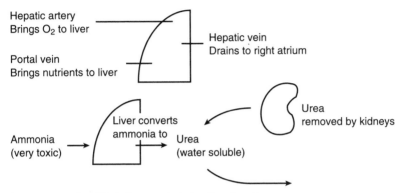

FIGURE 4-2 A simplified diagram depicting liver function.

ASCITES

Accumulation of fluid in the abdominal cavity, or ascites, is caused by decreased protein content and an increase in osmolarity. Pressure from the ascites frequently results in dyspnea. It is a common complication of advanced hepatic disease. Sodium restriction is the cornerstone of therapy, along with diuretics. Paracentesis (removal of fluid from the abdominal cavity) is rarely used because it may precipitate hepatic coma, shock, or hypovolemia (see Paracentesis).

BILIRUBIN

Bilirubin is the pigmented end product of hemoglobin breakdown and a component of bile. Bilirubin is normally excreted with bile into the duodenum, then it is broken down by bacteria in the lower intestines. When the hepatic or biliary ducts become blocked for any reason, bile is no longer excreted into the bowel. It is absorbed in the blood (causing jaundice) and excreted by the kidneys.

(continued)

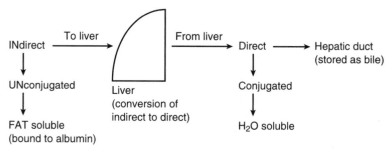

Figure 4-3 Bilirubin conversion.

Any increase in indirect bilirubin = liver disease (hepatitis or cirrhosis). Liver cannot convert bilirubin and it remains unchanged.

Any increase in direct bilirubin = biliary tract obstruction. Liver converts bilirubin, but obstruction is met; direct bilirubin accumulates.

Any increase in **both** direct and indirect bilirubin = hepatic failure.

BILROTH PROCEDURE (see Ulcers)

BLAKEMORE TUBE (see Sengstaken-Blakemore Tube)

BOWEL OBSTRUCTION (see also Colostomy, Ileostomy)

Bowel obstruction develops when intestinal contents cannot pass through the lumen of the bowel. It may be due to mechanical causes, neurogenic causes, or vascular abnormalities.

Types:

Simple: No interference with blood supply.

Strangulated: Blood supply decreased to obstructed segment; ischemia occurs; may progress to necrosis and gangrene.

Incarcerated: Blood supply severely altered. Necrosis, gangrene occur.

TABLE 4-1. Large Bowel versus Small Bowel Obstruction

Characteristic	Large Bowel	Small Bowel
Stool	None	Intermittent until bowel clears, then none
Distension	Pronounced	Minimal
Vomiting	Not common	Occurs if obstruction proximal to ileum
Pain	Mild, steady	Cramping in upper abdominal area

CECOSTOMY (see Colostomy)

CIRRHOSIS (see also Bilirubin)

Cirrhosis is a disease in which liver damage is followed by scarring, with fibrous tissue formation compressing blood, lymph, and bile channels. It is the final stage of many types of liver injury.

- **Portal cirrhosis (Laënnec's):** Associated with alcoholism. It is the most common type and has three components: (1) destruction of hepatic tissue, (2) diffuse increase in fibrous tissue, and (3) disorganized regeneration. The liver is enlarged and firm. An important secondary factor is the development of portal hypertension and esophageal or gastric varices (see Esophageal Varices).

- **Posthepatitic cirrhosis:** Associated with viral or toxic hepatitis. The liver is shrunken and irregular with large regeneration nodules and fibrous tissue.

- **Biliary cirrhosis:** Associated with intrahepatic cholestasis. There is scarring around the ducts and lobules, and there may be a disturbance of immune mechanisms.

COLITIS

Ulcerative colitis is an inflammatory disease of the colon with an unknown cause. In the early stages, only the rectum or rectosigmoid colon is affected, with the rectal mucosa containing many superficial bleeding points. As the disease progresses, the bowel mucosa becomes edematous and thickened. The superficial bleeding points enlarge and become ulcerated, causing the ulcers to bleed or perforate. The continuous healing process, with the formation of scar tissue between the frequent relapses, causes the colon to lose its normal elasticity and absorptive capability.

Treatment is directed toward combating infection, reducing the motility of the inflamed bowel, and restoring nutrition. Approximately 20% of patients require surgery for a subtotal colectomy and ileostomy due to hemorrhage or perforation.

COLOSTOMY (see also Bowel Obstruction, Ileostomy)

Colostomy is the opening of some portion of colon to the abdominal surface. It is named for the section of the colon cut into.

Sigmoid and Descending Colostomy

Stoma is normally in left area of colon. Rectum, anus, and damaged portion of large intestine are removed. Elimination is fecal material. Surgery is permanent; prognosis is good.

(continued)

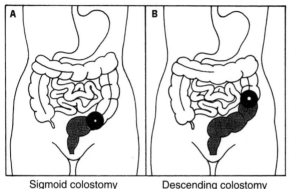

Sigmoid colostomy   Descending colostomy

Figure 4-4 Sigmoid and descending colostomy. *Shaded area* indicates section of bowel removed.

Transverse Colostomy

Stoma is usually slightly above and to one side of navel. Only damaged portion of large intestine is removed. It usually is a "resting" process with closure later. Management can be with irrigation, which gives 50% control (stays clean 6 to 10 hours). Two types of colostomy, performed along the transverse colon, are:

Double Barrel Transverse Colostomy

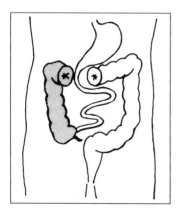

Figure 4-5 Double barrel transverse colostomy. (Courtesy of United Ostomy Association, Irvine, CA.)

There are two stomas, one active, one inactive. Active stoma diverts feces to outside (bypassing injury or inflammation), and inactive stoma drains mucous until healing is complete. It requires constant wearing of an appliance. Ostomy is usually closed within 6 months and the bowel is rejoined.

(continued)

Loop Transverse Colostomy

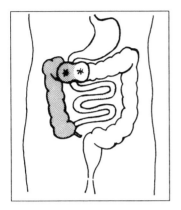

FIGURE 4-6 Loop colostomy. (Courtesy of United Ostomy Association, Irvine, CA.)

Intact loop of bowel is brought through abdomen and held in place by plastic bridge or anchor. It is temporary for as little as 10 days or as long as 9 months.

Ascending Colostomy (Cecostomy)

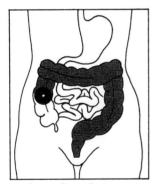

Ascending colostomy

FIGURE 4-7 Ascending colostomy. *Shaded area* indicates section of bowel removed.

Stoma is in right lower quadrant. It functions like an ileostomy, as elimination is thin and filled with gastric juices. Flow is constant and requires constant wearing of an appliance. Surgery is temporary.

NOTES

CULLEN'S SIGN (see also Pancreatitis)

Ecchymosis around umbilicus, or Cullen's sign, is associated with severe intraperitoneal hemorrhage.

REMEMBER:

> C· ← umbilicus   "C" shape for Cullen's

DIVERTICULITIS

A diverticulum of the colon is an outpouching of mucosa through a weak point in the muscular layer of the bowel wall. It generally results from persistent and abnormally high intracolonic pressure. The presence of many diverticula in the sigmoid and the ascending colon is called diverticulosis. If diverticula become inflamed, the term diverticulitis is used. The cause is unknown, with at least 10% of the middle-aged population being affected. No treatment is necessary for diverticula causing no symptoms; however, symptomatic diverticula generally require medical therapy. A possible complication is perforation with resultant abscess formation or generalized peritonitis. The inflammatory process may also cause bowel obstruction, and the patient may require surgery. Occasionally, a portion of the involved bowel is removed and a colostomy is placed.

(continued)

NOTES

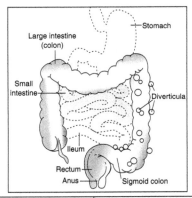

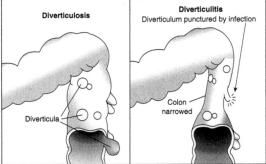

FIGURE 4-8 (*Top*) Location of diverticula in the sigmoid colon. (*Bottom left*) Diverticulosis. (*Bottom right*) Diverticulitis. (National Digestive Diseases Information Clearinghouse. [1989]. *Clearinghouse fact sheet: Diverticulosis and diverticulitis.* NIH publication no. 90–1163. Washington, DC: US Department of Health and Human Services.)

◖ DOBHOFF FEEDING TUBE*

Points to remember regarding insertion:

• Be sure to activate the hydromer lubricant on weighted tip of tube by dipping the tip in water.

• Passage can be facilitated by the use of the "flow-through" stylet. For stylet placement, inject approximately 10 cc of water into the tube to activate the hydromer lubricant coating. Insert the stylet fully into the feeding tube and pass through nostril. Once the feeding tube with the stylet has been inserted into the patient, **do not** pull the stylet back

(*continued*)

---

*Note: Some institutions do not allow RNs to pass any enteral tubes requiring a stylet.

and forth to manipulate it within the tube. (This avoids damage or puncture of the lung, should the tube be in the tracheobronchial tree.)

• Confirm placement of tube before removing stylet.

• Spontaneous transpyloric passage of the weighted tip often occurs within 24 to 48 hours.

DUODENAL ULCER (see Ulcers)

ENCEPHALOPATHY, LIVER

Encephalopathy is a disorder characterized by an increase in the blood ammonia level (the liver is no longer available to remove it by converting it to urea). Any increase in the ammonia level results in a toxic effect on the brain, and the patient exhibits impaired mentation, neuromuscular disturbance, and an altered level of consciousness. Encephalopathy can be precipitated by diuretics, acute infection, increased protein, elevated BUN, or GI bleeding in patients with renal disease.

TABLE 4-2. Stages of Liver Encephalopathy

Stage	Impairment
I	Slight personality change; impaired mentation
II	Mental confusion; asterixis (hands "flap")
III	Lethargic
IV	Unresponsive (high mortality)

Treatment:

• Restrict protein in diet

• Administer oral neomycin (alters gut flora so blood is not broken down and changed to ammonia)

• Administer lactulose (promotes ammonia secretion)

• Peritoneal dialysis or liver transplant may be necessary

• Monitor potassium levels (kidneys retain ammonium ions along with potassium ions)

• Do not administer lactated Ringer's via IV (diseased liver converts this to lactic acid and produces more ammonia)

ESOPHAGEAL VARICES (see also Cirrhosis, Sengstaken-Blakemore Tube, Shunts)

In a scarred, cirrhotic liver, the intrahepatic veins may be squeezed shut so that blood backs up into the portal vein and into diverting channels

(continued)

around the esophagus, causing the life-threatening complication of varices. Restoration of blood volume and control of bleeding are the immediate aim of treatment.

◯ GASTRECTOMY (see Ulcers)

◯ GASTRIC pH

Use Nitrazine paper (phenaphthazine) for pH determination. Apply several drops of NG aspirate to paper and shake off excess. Read **immediately** from comparison chart on side of dispenser. Remember, Nitrazine paper becomes inactive if it becomes wet from other fluids. If the gastric contents have antacids in them, flush NG with saline and reaspirate.

Normal pH is 4.5 to 7.5. Usual treatment for pH 5.0 or below is with antacid (Maalox).

◯ GASTRIC ULCER (see Ulcers)

◯ GASTROINTESTINAL BLEEDING (see also Sengstaken-Blakemore Tube, Transjugular Intrahepatic Portosystemic Shunt)

Upper GI bleeds may be due to:
- Duodenal or gastric ulcer, erosive gastritis
- Esophageal varices, esophagitis, esophageal tear
- Tumors, occasionally

Lower GI bleeds may be due to:
- Ruptured diverticulum
- Ischemic bowel
- Polyps, tumors, occasionally
- Ulcerative colitis
- Eroding aortic aneurysm

REMEMBER, **the rapidity of the blood loss is often more important than the amount.**

Treatment involves replacing lost fluid and controlling bleeding with ice lavage, a Sengstaken-Blakemore tube, and/or IV Pitressin. Sclerotherapy or variceal banding is indicated for small varices and a TIPS procedure (transjugular intahepatic portosystemic shunt) for large varices.

◯ GASTROJEJUNOSTOMY (see Ulcers)

GREY TURNER'S SIGN

Grey Turner's sign is bluish color of the flank due to retroperitoneal bleeding.

GUAIAC TEST (see Hemoccult Test)

HEMOCCULT TEST

This qualitative test is performed to detect fecal occult blood.

1. Collect a small fecal sample on one end of the applicator.

2. Apply a thin smear inside Box A of Hemoccult slide.

3. Reuse the applicator to obtain a second sample from a different part of the stool. Apply a thin smear inside Box B of same slide.

4. Close the cover.

5. If testing immediately, wait 3 to 5 minutes before developing. Otherwise, store slides as directed for up to 14 days until ready to develop.

6. Open the flap in the back of the slide and apply two drops of Hemoccult developer to the guaiac paper directly over each smear.

7. Read results within 60 seconds. Any trace of blue on or at the edge of the smear is positive for occult blood.

REMEMBER:

• Ascorbic acid (vitamin C) can cause false negative result if >250 mg/ day is ingested.

• Some fecal samples have a high bile content that causes them to appear blue-green in the test area. Test results are positive only if additional blue is formed **after** developer is added.

• Slides and developer have expiration dates.

HEPATIC FAILURE (see also Bilirubin)

Liver is unable to conjugate bilirubin with hepatic failure, and an increase in both indirect and direct bilirubin is seen.

HEPATITIS

Hepatitis is the widespread inflammation of liver cells and edema, which leads to distortion of the liver's lobular shape. The liver becomes enlarged, exhibiting a smooth edge and tenderness on palpation.

(continued)

Hepatitis A (infectious hepatitis)

Hepatitis A can be transmitted by the fecal or oral route. Because the organism is also food and water borne, shellfish are often associated with transmission. Clinical course of infection is usually over 1 to 3 months, with a complete recovery. Enteric precautions should be maintained, although after the patient's jaundice disappears, he is no longer infectious.

Hepatitis B (serum hepatitis)

Hepatitis B can be transmitted via contact with blood or blood products, requiring a break in the skin for actual transmission to occur. Hepatitis B is the leading cause of fulminant liver failure. Isolation and enteric precautions are required. After the patient's jaundice subsides, isolation can be discontinued, although the patient is considered infectious as long as an antigen can be identified in the serum. (Approximately 4% of patients who have recovered from hepatitis B are still infectious after 6 months.) The patient is then considered a carrier.

Lab profile:

• SGOT, SGPT increase. Levels rise during prejaundice phase to peaks of >500 by the time jaundice appears, followed by a rapid fall over several days. SGOT, SGPT levels return to normal 2 to 5 weeks after onset of jaundice.

• Albumin is slightly decreased.

• Serum globulin is increased.

• Bile pigments are altered (see Bilirubin).

Treatment consists of a long period of rest, lactulose to promote ammonia secretion, and a decreased protein diet (protein breaks down in the GI tract to ammonia).

Hepatitis C (non-A, non-B)

Hepatitis C is caused by a virus found to be usually transmitted via blood, blood products, and shared needles, though there is some evidence that it may also be transmitted sexually. It has better prognosis than hepatitis B. The hepatitis C antibody does not confer immunity, and patients may progress to chronic infection.

⬤ HYPERALIMENTATION (see TPN)

⬤ ILEAL CONDUIT (Urostomy)

Ileal conduit is so called because the surgeon converts 6 to 8 inches of ileum into a conduit or "pipeline" for urinary drainage. The ureters are spliced into one end of conduit and brought out the other through the

(continued)

abdominal wall to form a stoma. Bowel is rejoined and continues to function normally; elimination through the stoma is urine. Patient has no voluntary control, with a few drops of urine discharging every 10 to 20 seconds.

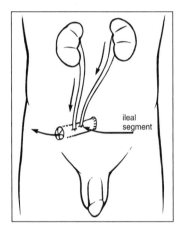

Figure 4-9 Ileal conduit.

ILEOSTOMY (see also Bowel Obstruction, Colostomy)

Ileostomy is the opening of the ileum onto the abdominal surface, usually performed for ulcerative colitis and sometimes for Crohn's disease or cancer of the bowel. The entire large intestine and rectum are removed (total colectomy). Discharge liquid flows constantly. The stoma is ½ to 1 inch long, usually formed to protrude so the discharge doesn't flow directly onto the skin.

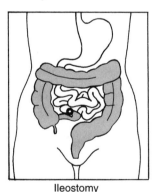

Ileostomy

Figure 4-10 Ileostomy. *Shaded area* indicates section removed.

KEHR'S SIGN

Kehr's sign is left shoulder pain due to diaphragmatic irritation related to splenic rupture. An increase in WBCs is common.

◉ MALLORY-WEISS SYNDROME

Mallory-Weiss syndrome is painless GI hemorrhage related to weakness in the esophageal wall causing rupture during coughing or vomiting (or any increase in abdominal pressure).

◉ McBURNEY'S POINT

McBurney's point is located one-third the distance from the anterior superior iliac spine to the umbilicus. McBurney's sign is tenderness at the site and is associated with acute appendicitis.

◉ MESOCAVAL SHUNT (see Shunts)

◉ MURPHY'S SIGN

Murphy's sign is severe pain and inspiratory arrest with palpation of the right upper quadrant. It is indicative of cholecystitis.

◉ PANCREATITIS

Pancreatitis is an autodigestive disease related to escape of activated enzymes from acinar cells. About 60% of cases are related to alcoholism, 20% to biliary tract disease, and less than 10% to gallstones or posttraumatic injury to the pancreas.

Symptoms:
- Severe epigastric pain radiating to the back
- Abdominal distension, nausea, vomiting
- Absent bowel sounds
- Fatty, foul-smelling stools
- Increased serum amylase (2 to 3 days)
- Increased urine amylase (5 to 7 days)
- Increased lipase
- **No** rebound tenderness

The patient may also exhibit hypocalcemia (resulting in twitching and seizures), HHNK, bilateral rales, atelectasis of the left base, and a pleural effusion. ARDS is sometimes an end result, due to the enzymes released by the pancreas causing loss of surfactant.

(continued)

Hemorrhagic pancreatitis causes blood to pool retroperitoneally, producing a bluish color of the flank (Grey Turner's sign) and around the umbilicus (Cullen's sign).

Treatment:

• Demerol (**no** morphine, codeine, or hydromorphone [Dilaudid], because they cause spasms of sphincter of Oddi)

• Fluid replacement (for loss due to vomiting)

• Decrease pancreatic stimulation (by decreasing HCl in stomach; Tagamet, Zantac, Pepcid, Maalox, NPO)

• NG suction

• Possible peritoneal lavage

• Whipple procedure (removal of gallbladder, distal portion of stomach, duodenum, and head of pancreas. Remaining stomach, pancreas, and common bile duct are anastomosed to jejunum.)

• Long term: insulin dependence

PARACENTESIS

Paracentesis is a "tapping" of the abdomen by means of a hollow needle or trocar to draw off fluid. It is rarely used because the procedure can precipitate hepatic coma, shock, or hypovolemia. If the abdomen is tight with fluid and producing dyspnea, or if fluid samples are needed, the procedure may be necessary. Generally, only enough fluid is removed to make the patient comfortable. One liter of ascitic fluid contains as much protein as 200 mL of whole blood, thus salt-poor albumin is often given to counteract the loss. Other complications are hypovolemia (fluid shifts rapidly into the peritoneal cavity to replace what was lost) and reduced tissue perfusion (leading to decreased systemic circulation, renal failure, or hepatic coma).

PEPTIC ULCER (see Ulcers)

PERITONEAL LAVAGE

Peritoneal lavage is used for penetrating abdominal trauma, if surgical exploration is not indicated, or for blunt abdominal injury with altered pain response or unexplained hypovolemia in a multiple trauma victim.

(continued)

Procedure:

1. Bladder is emptied and NG inserted to decompress stomach.

2. Small 1- to 2-cm incision is made by physician between umbilicus and pubic symphysis.

3. Lactated Ringer's or normal saline, usually 1 liter, is then instilled by gravity, while turning patient side to side.

4. IV bag is dropped and fluid is allowed to drain passively.

5. Specimens sent to laboratory. Positive for bleeding (exact levels vary with institution) if:

   a. 10 to 20 mL of gross blood obtained on initial aspirate

   b. RBCs >100,000 mm^3

   c. WBCs >500 mm^3

   d. Presence of bacteria or fecal material

   e. Elevated amylase

PERITONITIS

An inflammatory involvement of the peritoneum, peritonitis is caused by trauma or by rupture of an organ containing bacteria, which are then introduced into the abdominal cavity. Some of the organisms commonly found are *E. coli,* streptococci (both aerobic and anaerobic), staphylococci, and pneumococci.

Treatment with massive doses of antibiotics to combat the infection is initiated, and attempts are made to restore intestinal motility by insertion of intestinal or gastric tubes. Fluids and electrolytes are replaced. If the peritonitis is caused by a perforation that is releasing irritating or infected material into the abdominal cavity, surgery to close the abnormal opening and remove the accumulated fluid is indicated.

PORTACAVAL SHUNT (see Shunts)

PSOAS SIGN

To elicit psoas sign, patient is asked to raise right leg with examiner's hand providing resistance just above the right knee. Alternately, the patient is turned to the left side and the right leg is extended at the hip by the examiner. Increased abdominal pain with either maneuver indicates a positive result, suggesting irritation of the psoas muscle by an inflamed appendix.

○ SENGSTAKEN-BLAKEMORE TUBE (see also Esophageal Varices, Shunts)

Sengstaken-Blakemore tube stops acute variceal hemorrhage 85% to 90% of the time. Scissors should be placed at the bedside as a precaution to allow rapid deflation of the esophageal balloon should the gastric balloon rupture (if not cut, tube would rise to the nasopharynx and obstruct the airway).

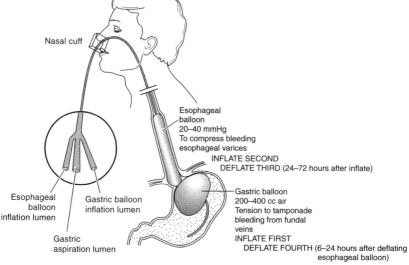

FIGURE 4-11 Sengstaken-Blakemore tube. (Adapted with permission from Ignatavicius, D. D., Workman, M. L., Mishler, M. A. [1995]. *Medical surgical nursing: A nursing process approach.* Vol. 2. [2nd ed.]. Philadelphia: WB Saunders.)

○ SHUNTS

- **Mesocaval shunt:** Anastomoses the superior mesenteric vein to the inferior vena cava.

- **Splenorenal (Warren) shunt:** Anastomoses the splenic vein to the left renal vein. Some hepatic flow is preserved, but thrombosis of the shunt is common.

- **Portacaval shunts:** Rarely used. It anastomoses the portal vein to the inferior vena cava. The problems arise from the fact that the liver is then unable to detoxify, and encephalopathy usually develops.

(continued)

- **TIPS (transjugular intrahepatic portosystem shunt):** Has largely replaced previous shunts. Total portal decompression is accomplished through the means of a functional "H" graft contained within the liver parenchyma, producing a side to side portosystemic shunt. Portal hypertension is reduced and bleeding esophageal varices are eliminated when flow is diverted from the portal vein into the inferior vena cava.

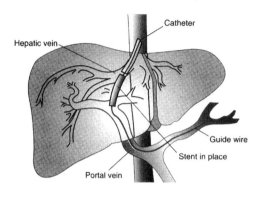

FIGURE 4-12 Transjugular intrahepatic portosystem shunt (TIPS). A stent is inserted through a catheter to the portal vein to divert blood flow and reduce portal hypertension.

SPLENORENAL SHUNT (see Shunts)

TIPS (see Shunts)

TPN (Total Parenteral Nutrition)

Total parenteral nutrition is administration of complete nutrition by IV infusion of amino acids and a non-nitrogen caloric source (dextrose), together with electrolytes, vitamins, and minerals.

REMEMBER:

- An infusion pump is mandatory for best control of the infusion rate.
- TPN bags routinely contain >1000 mL, and therefore it is appropriate to change a bag before it is completely empty. Never attempt to "catch up" by increasing the rate or, likewise, slowing the rate.
- With each new bag, tubing and filter should be changed.
- A central line port should be dedicated to TPN and **never** used to monitor CVP, take blood samples, or administer blood or IV fluids. Consider it the patient's "life line."
- If the next bag of TPN is unavailable at the scheduled time, start D10W in the interim.

(continued)

- Patient should be scheduled for frequent, routine D-sticks and have daily weights done.

Complications of TPN:

- Technical complications include pneumothorax, subclavian artery injury, air embolism.

- Metabolic abnormalities include increased or decreased glucose, increased or decreased potassium, and possible hypophosphatemia.

- Septic events can occur related to catheter sepsis or contamination of the TPN solution.

TRANSJUGULAR INTRAHEPATIC PORTOSYSTEMIC SHUNT (see Shunts)

TUBE FEEDINGS

TABLE 4-3. Therapeutic Equivalents for Tube Feedings

Equivalent	Supplement
1 kcal/cc lactose-free	Osmolite HN
	Isocal HN
	Entrition HN
1.5 kcal/cc lactose-free (flavored)	Ensure Plus
	Comply
	Nutren 1.5
	Sustacal HC
2 kcal/cc lactose-free	Two-Cal HN
	Isocal HCN
	Nutren 2.0
	Magnacal
1 kcal/cc lactose-free with fiber	Enrich
	Jevity
	Vitaneed
	Profiber
	Complete modified Sustacal with fiber
Low residue	Vital High Nitrogen
High nitrogen	Criticare HN
Low fat	Pepti-2000
	Vivonex T.E.N.
Protein module	Promod
	Propac
Carbohydrate module	Polycose powder or liquid
Fat module	Corn oil (obtained from dietary department)

⬤ ULCERATIVE COLITIS (see Colitis)

⬤ ULCERS

Peptic ulcers are acute or chronic ulcerations occurring in a portion of the digestive tract that is in contact with gastric secretions. Duodenal ulcers comprise about 80% of ulcers, with gastric ulcers comprising 20%.

Duodenal ulcers occur in about 10% of the population and are related to an increased quantity or increased level of acidity of the gastric juice. Although they do not become malignant, perforation is common. Surgical measures are indicated only after a thorough trial of conservative measures and medical management. Current practice is to perform a gastric resection with a vagotomy to eliminate the acid secreting stimulus to gastric cells. The branches of the vagus nerve are severed, the number of which depends on how much reduction in secretory ability is desired. If an insufficient number are cut, however, the ability of the stomach to secrete regenerates with time and then requires further intervention.

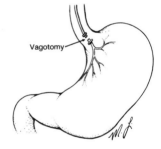

Vagotomy

FIGURE 4-13 Vagotomy.

Gastric ulcers are similar in many respects to duodenal ulcers, but they are not associated with an accumulation of increased acid. Rather, gastric ulcers reabsorb the excess acid being secreted through the mucous membrane by abnormal diffusion of H^+. This diffusion results in a damaged mucous barrier and renders the ulcer likely to bleed. Treatment is usually aggressive because about 10% of gastric ulcers prove to be malignant, and a resection is performed via a Bilroth I procedure (partial gastrectomy with a gastroduodenoscopy; distal one-third to one-half of the stomach is excised with remaining portion anastomosed to duodenum) or a Bilroth II procedure (partial gastrectomy with a gastrojejunostomy; distal segment of the stomach and antrum are removed with anastomoses of the remainder to the jejunum and closing of the duodenal stump).

(continued)

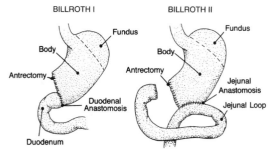

BILLROTH I

BILLROTH II

Fundus

Body

Antrectomy

Duodenal
Anastomosis

Duodenum

Fundus

Body

Antrectomy

Jejunal
Anastomosis

Jejunal Loop

FIGURE 4-14 Billroth I and II procedures.

URETEROSTOMY

Ureters are disengaged from the bladder and brought through the abdominal wall at waist level in a ureterostomy. Sometimes two stomas (one on each side) or one ureter is anastomosed to the other and brought to the skin surface to form a single stoma. Elimination is urine and requires the constant wearing of an appliance.

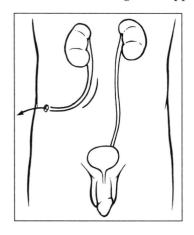

FIGURE 4-15 Cutaneous ureterostomy.

URINARY CATHETERS

Catheters may be self-retaining (able to maintain themselves in cavities) or non-self-retaining (must be secured with tape if left indwelling). They come in various sizes, graded from 14 French (smallest) to 22 French (largest), and in various shapes, with the curved tip frequently used for males and the straight tip for females. The self-retaining protuberance at the tip of the Malecot and de Pezzer catheters must be elongated with a stylet, which is passed through the lumen before insertion. After insertion,

(continued)

the stylet is removed and the protuberance secures the catheter in place. Straight catheters may have a single eye or many eyes, and they may have a round tip or a whistle tip.

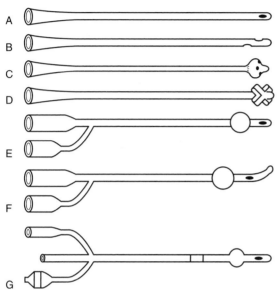

FIGURE 4-16 Different types of commonly used catheters. **(A and B)** Simple urethral catheters; **(C)** mushroom or de Pezzer; **(D)** winged-tip or Malecot; **(E)** Foley with inflated retention bag; **(F)** Foley with Coude tip; and **(G)** 3-way catheter (in this illustration the third lumen opens into the urethra to permit irrigation; usually opens at tip for irrigation of the bladder).

⬤ **URINARY DIVERSION** (see Ileal Conduit, Ureterostomy)

⬤ **UROSTOMY** (see Ileal Conduit)

⬤ **VAGOTOMY** (see Ulcers)

⬤ **WHIPPLE PROCEDURE** (see Pancreatitis)

PART
5
Renal System

 ACUTE RENAL FAILURE

Acute renal failure is the rapid deterioration of renal function with high blood concentration of nitrogen waste products. There are three major categories:

Prerenal (hypoperfused kidney)

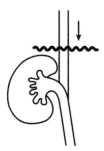

FIGURE 5-1 Hypoperfused kidney.

Prerenal events occur before blood reaches the kidney, leading to renal hypoperfusion and resulting in decrease of glomerular perfusion, CHF, and low blood pressure. This is the most common cause of acute renal failure.

Intrarenal (diseased kidney)

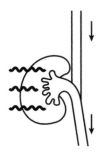

FIGURE 5-2 Diseased kidney.

(continued)

Intrarenal failure is due to intrinsic damage to the kidney. There are two types:

- *Glomerulonephritis* has an immunologic basis and causes change in the glomerular membrane and/or cellular structure. The glomerulus loses its ability to be semipermeable, and protein and RBCs pass through into the urine, resulting in hematuria and proteinuria.
- *Acute tubular necrosis* has two origins:

1. Ischemic (oliguric) necrosis is related to catastrophic hypotension from many sources, for example, surgery, cardiac or septic shock, trauma, hemorrhage. It is more serious than nephrotoxic necrosis because cells are destroyed in a layer than can't regenerate (the "basement membrane").

2. Nephrotoxic (nonoliguric) necrosis is related to environmental or occupational insults to the kidney, for example, large doses of iatrogenic agents such as gentamicin, amikacin, carbenicillin. It has a good prognosis for recovery because the damage involves only the tubule's layer of epithelial cells, which can regenerate.

TABLE 5-1. Use of Laboratory Values in Differentiating Acute Tubular Necrosis from Decreased Renal Perfusion

Test	Acute Tubular Necrosis	Reduced Renal Blood Flow
URINE		
Volume	<400 mL/24 h	<400 mL/24 h
Sodium	>40 mEq/L	<5 mEq/L
Specific gravity	1.010	Usually >1.020
Osmolality	250–350 mOsm/L	Usually >400 mOsm/L
Urea	200–300 mg/100 mL	Usually >600 mg/100 mL
Creatinine	<60 mg/100 mL	Usually >150 mg/100 mL
Fe_{Na}	>3.0%	<1.0%
BLOOD		
BUN:Cr	10:1	Usually >20:1
RESPONSES TO		
Mannitol	None	None or flow increases to >40 mL/h
Furosemide	None	Flow increases to >40 mL/h

Fe_{Na}, fractional excretion of sodium; BUN, blood urea nitrogen; Cr, blood urea nitrogen–creatinine ratio

(*continued*)

NOTES

Postrenal (obstructed kidney)

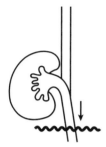

FIGURE 5-3 Obstructed kidney.

Postrenal failure is due to blockage of flow in the urinary tract. Treatment of acute renal failure in the first 24 to 48 hours includes correcting hypotension or fluid deficits, administering furosemide (Lasix) (80 to 320 mg initial dose) or mannitol (12.5 to 25 g), and/or giving a trial of low-dose dopamine (1 to 3 μg/kg/min) plus Lasix.

☐ ACUTE TUBULAR NECROSIS (ATN) (see Acute Renal Failure)

☐ ADH (Antidiuretic Hormone) (see also Renin-Angiotensin System)

ADH is controlled by osmoreceptors (sensitive to osmolar change) and baroreceptors (sensitive to pressure change). Normally, osmoreceptors in the hypothalamus stimulate the posterior pituitary to release ADH in response to a rise in serum osmolality (ie, when water is lost). ADH then acts on the renal tubule to increase water permeability, and water is reabsorbed. The reverse is true: when serum osmolality falls (water is retained), excess water is excreted by the kidney.

Baroreceptors influence ADH release in pathologic states. When blood volume is down about 10% or the blood pressure falls, these receptors in the heart and various blood vessels contract and initiate a stimulus for ADH release. Water is then retained by the kidney. The reverse is true when baroreceptors are stretched more than normal (ie, when blood volume rises).

Baroreceptors override osmoreceptors. For example, if blood volume is low, water is retained even though the osmolality drops. This is a protective mechanism whereby the body attempts to maintain blood volume even though hemodilution results.

◐ ALDOSTERONE (see also ADH, Renin-Angiotensin System)

Aldosterone is released by the adrenal cortex in response to angiotensin II, causing sodium and water to be reabsorbed and potassium and hydrogen to be excreted.

REMEMBER: Because aldosterone causes sodium **and** water to be saved, the actual concentration of sodium does **not** change, only the extracellular volume.

Aldosterone is released for:
- Increased potassium (to decrease the K^+ level)
- Decreased sodium (to save Na^+)
- Hypovolemia (to save H_2O)

No aldosterone is released in cases of:
- Increased sodium (to decrease the Na^+ level)
- Decreased potassium (to save K^+)

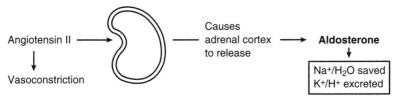

Angiotensin II ⟶ Causes adrenal cortex to release ⟶ **Aldosterone**

Vasoconstriction

Na^+/H_2O saved
K^+/H^+ excreted

FIGURE 5-4 Aldosterone release.

◐ ANATOMY, RENAL

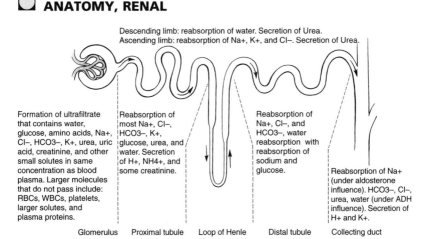

Descending limb: reabsorption of water. Secretion of Urea.
Ascending limb: reabsorption of Na+, K+, and Cl–. Secretion of Urea.

Formation of ultrafiltrate that contains water, glucose, amino acids, Na+, Cl–, HCO3–, K+, urea, uric acid, creatinine, and other small solutes in same concentration as blood plasma. Larger molecules that do not pass include: RBCs, WBCs, platelets, larger solutes, and plasma proteins.

Reabsorption of most Na+, Cl–, HCO3–, K+, glucose, urea, and water. Secretion of H+, NH4+, and some creatinine.

Reabsorption of Na+, Cl–, and HCO3–, water reabsorption with reabsorption of sodium and glucose.

Reabsorption of Na+ (under aldosterone influence). HCO3–, Cl–, urea, water (under ADH influence). Secretion of H+ and K+.

Glomerulus   Proximal tubule   Loop of Henle   Distal tubule   Collecting duct

FIGURE 5-5 Functions in each portion of the nephron.

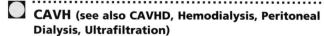

CAVH (see also CAVHD, Hemodialysis, Peritoneal Dialysis, Ultrafiltration)

Continuous arteriovenous hemofiltration is the filtration of blood at mild pressure, convectively removing plasma water with dissolved micromolecular components while retaining formed elements, proteins, and other elements larger than the clearance range of the membrane.

Advantages

- Control of fluid balance with high rate of fluid removed.
- Ease of hourly replacement (as opposed to hemodialysis, which causes drastic fluid changes).
- Virtually no risk of air embolism.
- No special machines or equipment.

Disadvantages

- Requires anticoagulation for patency.
- Only minimal amounts of protein can be removed.
- Does not utilize diffusion (as does hemodialysis), and therefore, any BUN that is removed is due to convective transport. Accordingly, the removal of BUN is slow and very dependent on good blood flow through the filter (requires a mean arterial pressure of >60 mmHg).

Procedure

The hemofilter is connected directly to a suitable artery and vein (commonly the femoral or brachial). Heparin is infused in the arterial line at approximately 100 U/kg/hr. Substitution fluid is infused into the venous line at a rate sufficient to obtain either weight balance or desired amount of fluid withdrawal.

(*continued*)

NOTES

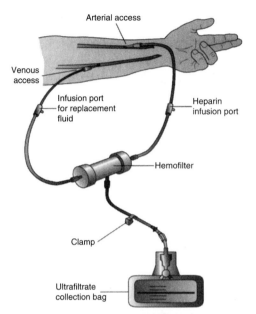

FIGURE 5-6 A schematic representation of a continuous arteriovenous hemofiltration (CAVH) system.

⬤ **CAVHD (see also CAVH, Hemodialysis, Peritoneal Dialysis, Ultrafiltration)**

Continuous arteriovenous hemofiltration dialysis combines the advantages of CVH with the filtering properties of dialysis. A dialysate solution is infused along with the hemofiltered blood. It is indicated for patients with catabolic acute renal failure and those hemodynamically unstable with azotemia.

⬤ **CONTINUOUS ARTERIOVENOUS HEMOFILTRATION (see CAVH)**

⬤ **CONTINUOUS ARTERIOVENOUS HEMOFILTRATION DIALYSIS (see CAVHD)**

NOTES

◯ CREATININE CLEARANCE

Creatinine clearance measures the efficiency of the glomerular filtration of plasma.

$$\text{Creatinine clearance} = \frac{140 - \text{age (yr)} \times \text{body weight (kg)}}{72 \times \text{serum creatinine}}$$

Normal:

Males: 107 to 139 mL/min

Females: 87 to 107 mL/min

◯ ERYTHROPOIETIN

Erythropoietin stimulates the production of RBCs in bone marrow and prolongs the life of the RBC. Kidneys either produce erythropoietin or they synthesize an enzyme that catalyzes its formation. The stimulation for production is believed to be decreased oxygen delivery to the kidney. A deficiency of erythropoietin is the primary cause of anemia in chronic renal failure.

◯ GLOMERULAR FILTRATION RATE

A clinical assessment tool, glomerular filtration rate (GFR) is used to determine renal function. The glomerulus (a capillary bed) filters about 120 to 125 mL/min through its membrane, or about 180 liters daily. The filtrate that results forms the main component of urine. Normal urine volume is approximately 1 liter per day; this indicates >99% reabsorption of filtrate. The glomerular filtration rate helps measure the degree of renal function. It is inversely related to creatinine.

Normal	125 mL/min
Renal insufficiency	<100 mL/min
Signs and symptoms of renal failure	<20 mL/min
Life-threatening renal failure	<10 mL/min

◯ GLOMERULONEPHRITIS (see Acute Renal Failure)

◯ HEMODIALYSIS (see also CAVH, CAVHD, Peritoneal Dialysis, Quinton Catheter, Ultrafiltration)

Hemodialysis is an extracorporeal technique for removing waste products or toxic substances from systemic circulation using a fistula, graft, or shunt. Principles are the same as for peritoneal dialysis.

(continued)

- **Fistula:** An anastomosis of an artery and a vein.

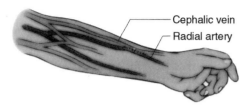

Cephalic vein
Radial artery

FIGURE 5-7 An internal arteriovenous fistula is created by a side-to-side anastomosis of the artery and vein.

- **Graft:** The connection of an artery and a vein from an autogenous vein (usually the saphenous) or a bovine or Gore-Tex graft.

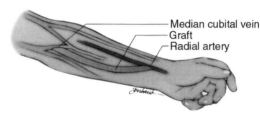

Median cubital vein
Graft
Radial artery

FIGURE 5-8 A graft can be established between the artery and vein.

- **Shunt:** An older form of the graft. It is an external connection of an artery and vein by means of a silicone Teflon connector. The main disadvantage (and danger) is disconnection of the shunt, resulting in hemorrhage, and it is therefore rarely used anymore.

Graft or Fistula Care

1. Auscultate bruit or palpate thrill to assess patency.

2. Do not perform venipuncture, start IV, give injections, or take BP with cuff on access arm.

Heparinization

Prior to procedure, "regional" heparinization is usually done to keep blood anticoagulated in the dialysis machine. Heparin rebound may occur for up to 10 hours after heparin has stopped. Monitor patient closely for bleeding.

HEMOFILTRATION (see CAVH)

HYPERCALCEMIA

- **Normal:** 8.5 to 10 mg/dL. Inversely related to PO_4.

It is difficult to identify specific signs and symptoms as being due exclusively to increased calcium, because so many are common to other

(continued)

disease states: lethargy, anorexia, nausea, vomiting, constipation, dehydration. Hypercalcemia often occurs in multiple myeloma (related to lesions releasing calcium into the plasma), vitamin D overdose, Paget's disease, and other skeletal diseases.

Treatment

• Provide adequate hydration (to decrease the risk of renal damage) with normal saline (to produce saline diuresis); fluids up to 200 cc/hr followed with Lasix 40 mg IV every 4 hours (no thiazides).

• Administer phosphates (to promote calcium deposition in bone and decrease absorption from GI tract).

• Administer corticosteroids, plicamycin (Mithramycin) (to lower serum calcium).

 HYPERKALEMIA

▪ **Normal:** 3.5 to 5.0 mEq/L.

Mild increase	5–6 mEq/L
Moderate increase	6–7 mEq/L
Severe increase (can result in cardiac arrest)	>7 mEq/L

Hyperkalemia is usually seen in patients with renal failure (no normal Na^+/K^+ exchange), hemorrhagic shock, Addison's disease (absence of aldosterone leads to heavy excretion of Na^+ and H_2O, leaving buildup of K^+), or massive cell damage (burns, MI, crushing injury).

Signs and Symptoms

• Prolonged PR, wide QRS, tall tented T
• Ascending muscle weakness (legs to trunk)
• Lethargy

Treatment

• Best treatment is to avoid the problem in the first place. *REMEMBER:* Renal patients require a low-potassium diet. ACE inhibitors cause K^+ retention.

• Administer glucose and insulin to drive the K^+ back into the cells.

• Give $NaHCO_3$ to correct the underlying metabolic acidosis.

• Give Kayexalate enema: 15 to 50 g in 100 to 200 mL of 20% sorbitol. Repeat every 3 hours until diarrhea produced.

• Peritoneal dialysis or hemodialysis may be indicated.

⬛ HYPERNATREMIA

- **Normal:** 135 to 145 mEq/L.

Hypernatremia occurs when H_2O losses exceed Na^+ losses or when H_2O intake is inadequate. It usually reflects in dehydration and results in hyperosmolality. Over time, an actual gain in Na^+ is seen, as in hyperaldosteronism.

Signs and Symptoms

- Thirst; dry, sticky mucous membranes
- Flushed skin, fever
- Oliguria
- Plasma osmolality >1.5 mOsm/L
- Urine specific gravity <1.015 if H_2O loss is nonrenal

Treatment

- Administer salt-free solutions (usually D5W) until level returns to normal, then ½ NS to avoid overcorrection. Be aware that the brain generates organic osmoles and "sucks up" aggressive fluid measures, producing cerebral edema. Also, think of rhabdomyolysis in a patient who has been "down" for a long period of time (see Rhabdomyolysis).

⬛ HYPERPHOSPHATEMIA

- **Normal:** 2.5 to 5.0 mg/dL.

Hyperphosphatemia is related to acute or chronic renal failure (kidney can't excrete), hypoparathyroidism.

Signs and Symptoms

- Cramps to tetany; similar to hypocalcemia

Treatment

- Administer aluminum hydroxide gels to bind phosphate and reduce serum levels
- Consider administration of acetazolamide (Diamox) to produce mild diuresis
- Dialysis may be indicated

⬛ HYPOCALCEMIA (see also Hypoparathyroid in Part 6, Endocrine System)

- **Normal:** 8.5 to 10 mg/dL

Hypocalcemia is related to chronic renal failure, multiple blood transfusions, excessive GI losses secondary to diarrhea or the effect of diuretics,

(continued)

or malabsorption syndromes. Because about 56% of serum calcium is bound to serum protein (and is therefore chemically inactive), any change in serum protein (as in renal disease) changes the total serum calcium (about 0.8 mg/dL of Ca^+ for each 1 g/dL change in albumin). The calcium value must be "corrected." For example:

Patient = serum calcium 9.0 with albumin 4.0 (normal 3.5–5 g/dL)
Later   = serum calcium 9.0 with albumin 1.0 g/dL

Formula for correction:

Multiply change in albumin (3.0) × 0.8 (constant) = 2.4 mg/dL Ca^+
Add result (2.4) to new Ca^+ value (9.0) = **11.4 mg/dL Ca^+**

The significance is that the patient's original lab test indicates a normal calcium, when in actuality *the patient is hypercalcemic* (see Hypercalcemia).

Signs and Symptoms

- Chvostek's and Trousseau's signs positive (see Part 1, Neurologic System)
- Seizures
- Laryngeal stridor (related to neuromuscular irritability)
- Bleeding abnormalities
- Prolonged QT interval

Treatment

- IV administration of a Ca^+ salt, usually 10% calcium gluconate or calcium chloride.

◨ HYPOKALEMIA

- **Normal:** 3.5 to 5.0 mEq/L.

Hypokalemia is seen in patients with loss of body fluids (diuresis, excess vomiting, colitis, gastric damage, gastric suction, vomiting, etc), adrenal disorders (aldosteronism, Cushing's disease, stress), CHF, or licorice candy addiction (glyceric acid has aldosterone-like effect).

Signs and Symptoms

- Disturbed mental function
- Speech changes
- Cardiac dysrhythmias, flattened T wave, present U wave
- Rapid weak pulse
- Decreased blood pressure

(*continued*)

Treatment
- Provide K^+ replacement (be careful in patients with renal insufficiency).

● HYPOMAGNESEMIA

- **Normal:** 1.5 to 2.5 mEq/L.

Hypomagnesemia frequently coexists with hypocalcemia and hypokalemia and is especially endemic to the ICU population. If the low calcium and potassium do not respond to treatment, it is more than likely related to the low magnesium, as magnesium interferes with K^+ replacement. Most hypomagnesemia disorders result from impaired absorption, excessive renal excretion, or fluid loss.

Signs and Symptoms
- Flushing, sweating
- Weak or absent deep tendon reflexes

Treatment
- Change in diet alone will usually correct a mild deficiency, or may require oral administration of magnesium salts.

- For a life-threatening deficiency, magnesium is added to IV solutions with an IV infusion rate not to exceed 150 mg/min. It is contraindicated in patients with renal insufficiency. Calcium gluconate reverses magnesium overdose.

● HYPONATREMIA

- **Normal:** 135 to 145 mEq/L.
- **Severe decrease:** <120 mEq/L.

With hyponatremia, the amount of Na^+ in extracellular compartments is deficient as compared with H_2O. It is related to:
- *Water intoxication*
- *Dilution* (related to expansion of total body H_2O) as with CHF, renal failure, cirrhosis, SIADH
    Treatment: Restrict intake (do not give hypertonic saline)
- *True hyponatremia* (low body Na^+) is related to burns, diarrhea, vomiting, adrenal insufficiency, drainage from fistulas, and so forth

Signs and Symptoms
- Weakness, irritability
- Weight loss or edema and weight gain

(continued)

- Decreased blood pressure
- Decreased skin turgor
- Tremors, convulsions
- Serum osmolality decreased with retention; increased with diuresis
- Urine specific gravity <1.010 with diuresis; >1.010 with water retention

Treatment

Administer normal saline at rapid rate (150 cc/hr); give Lasix 20 mg via IV every 4 hours; run serial labs. However, if the patient is hyponatremic secondary to SIADH, IV saline can worsen the condition. If patient is having seizures, 3% saline infusion may be considered (see Hot Salt in Part 8, Drugs, Doses, Tables). There are potentially disastrous consequences of both living with hyponatremia and treating it. Caution is the watchword.

 OSMOLALITY

A value used in clinical practice (more often than osmolarity), osmolality is expressed in milliosmoles per kg of water (mOsm/kg). It reflects the measurement of solute concentration *per kilogram* in blood and urine, and it is usually used when referring to fluids *inside* the body.

- **Normal:** 280 to 295 mOsm/kg.
- **Fluid overload:** <275 mOsm/kg.
- **Dehydration:** >295 mOsm/kg.

Serum osmolality is essentially what keep the fluids in their appropriate compartments, and it measures the "pulling power" of water. Na^+ accounts for at least half of this pulling power; each mEq of Na^+ equals one milliosmole. Therefore, $\frac{1}{2} \times 300 = 150$; and Na^+ normal is 135 to 145 mEq/L.

REMEMBER: Because sodium accounts for nearly half of the osmolality value, a quick way to do a rough guesstimate is to **multiply the Na^+ value by 2.**

Other things that account for osmolality:

- Amount of urea in plasma
- Amount of glucose in plasma
- Amount of plasma proteins in plasma (fibrinogen, albumin, globulins)

Osmolality depends on the mechanism of osmosis, causing water to be drawn into the solution of high concentration (the cell) until the concentration of particles is equalized. Intracellular and extracellular osmolalities are always equal; their measurement tells about overall body hydration or how concentrated body fluids are.

⬤ OSMOLARITY

Osmolarity is a value expressed in milliosmoles *per liter* of solution (mOsm/L) and is used to describe the number of dissolved particles within a solution. It is generally used to describe fluids *outside* the body; however, because 1 liter of H_2O weighs 1 kg, the term osmolarity is often used interchangeably with osmolality.

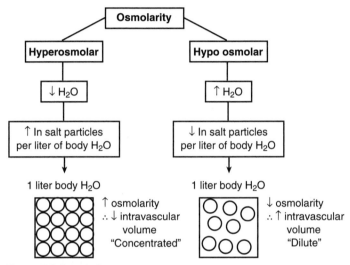

FIGURE 5-9 Osmolarity.

⬤ PERITONEAL DIALYSIS

Peritoneal dialysis is a method of dialysis in which the dialyzing fluid is instilled into the peritoneal cavity and the peritoneum serves as the dialyzing membrane. It is not as rapid as hemodialysis is for volume removal, nor does it provide as much plasma clearance. It's simplicity, however, makes it useful for hemodynamically unstable or bleeding patients.

Procedure

- Always use sterile technique.
- Bladder should be empty.
- Warm dialysate solution to body temperature. A solution too cool causes abdominal pain and cramping, whereas one too warm causes possible injury to the abdominal organs.

(continued)

• Weigh the patient before and after the procedure. Mark the midpoint of the abdomen with pen and also measure abdominal girth daily, using the same mark.

• Purge all air from the system by running the dialysate through the tubing. (A 1.5% solution is the most common choice, with 4.25% solution the second choice. Sometimes these two fluids are alternated during exchanges.)

• Add medication to the dialysate as prescribed (heparin, KCl, antibiotics, lidocaine).

• Infuse the dialysate as fast as tolerated, usually about 2 L in 6 to 15 minutes.

• The first exchange must be drained immediately to make sure the catheter is patent; all subsequent exchanges dwell according to physician orders, usually 20 to 45 minutes.

• Drain passively at end of dwell time, observing amount and characteristics of drainage:

    Normal = clear, pale yellow
    Cloudy = infection, peritonitis
    Brown = bowel perforation
    Amber = bladder perforation
    Bloody = common first to fourth exchange; if continues, may be abdominal bleeding

• After each exchange, record the infused volume, the dwell time, the total drainage, if patient is in a negative (patient giving up fluid) or positive (patient retaining fluid) balance, and cumulative balance.

Troubleshooting

• **If outflow stops or slows,** be sure clamp is open. Check tubing for kinks, turn patient side to side, or apply gentle pressure on abdomen to help get flow started.

• **If there is a sudden BP drop or tachycardia,** stop dialysis and notify physician.

• **Leakage at exit site** can be due to kinks in tubing. If tubing is OK, change dressing and wait for next exchange. If leak continues, be sure to weigh fluid loss on dressing and notify physician. Catheter may have slipped.

• **Sudden acute abdominal pain or back pain** may be related to the temperature of the solution. Also check for air in the system, and monitor the rate of infusion.

• **Scrotal swelling** is most likely due to a dislodged catheter. Notify the physician.

(continued)

PART 5 **RENAL SYSTEM** **207**

• **Muscle cramps and increased weakness** can be due to electrolyte imbalances. Send specimen to lab for electrolyte analysis.

◻ **QUINTON CATHETER (see also Hemodialysis)***

After new placement only: Using sterile technique, remove the heparin lock and flush the red port (arterial) and the blue port (venous) with 10 cc of normal saline. Flush forcefully while clamping down on insert site. Obtain chest x-ray film to confirm placement. Once confirmed, using 1000 U/cc heparin solution, flush the blue port (venous) with 1.3 cc and the red port (arterial) with 1.2 cc. No further flushing is permitted.

After the ports have been used for dialysis: Using sterile technique and a 1000 U/cc heparin solution, flush both the red and blue ports with 1.5 cc each.

Ports are **not** routinely flushed unless used.

* *This procedure is institution specific; it is suggested that individual hospital policy be reviewed.*

◻ **RENIN-ANGIOTENSIN SYSTEM (see also Aldosterone, ADH)**

Baroreceptors are the primary influence on sodium regulation. Located in the renal cortex, they control the release of renin from the adjacent cells (juxtaglomerular apparatus) in response to a decrease in blood pressure or a decrease in extracellular fluid. The renin converts angiotensin I to angiotensin II, a potent vasoconstrictor, which results in increased blood pressure and an increase in the GFR. Angiotensin II also triggers the release of aldosterone, causing an increase in renal sodium and water retention, thus increasing extracellular fluid volume, increasing blood pressure, and inhibiting further renin secretion. Any increase in Na^+ intake or an increase in blood volume also suppresses renin and aldosterone release, permitting an increase of Na^+ excretion.

(continued)

NOTES

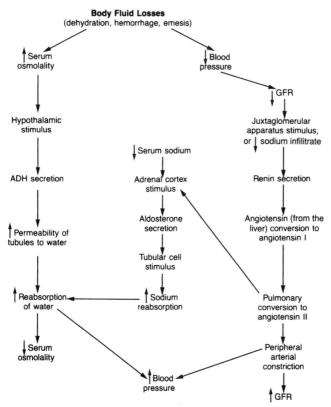

FIGURE 5-10 Relationship of antidiuretic hormone, renin, and aldosterone to fluid regulation by the kidneys.

RHABDOMYOLYSIS

Rhabdomyolysis occurs after skeletal muscle injury that allows the release of muscle cell contents (CK, LDH, myoglobin, uric acid, K^+, PO_4, organic acids, and creatinine) into extracellular fluid. Many of these contents are toxic at high levels, literally occluding the kidneys and causing renal failure. Trauma is the number one etiology, though often rhabdomyolysis is self-induced by healthy individuals who exceed their capacity for exercise endurance. Labs reveal an elevated serum CK, Hematest positive urine, and few or no RBCs on urinalysis. Treatment involves first flushing the kidneys with massive volume replacement and sometimes giving mannitol and Lasix concurrently for diuresis and to increase the serum osmolality.

ULTRAFILTRATION (see also CAVH, CAVHD, Hemodialysis, Peritoneal Dialysis)

Ultrafiltration is the process of removing excess H_2O in hemodialysis by creating a pressure differential between the blood and fluid compartments. The addition of positive pressure in the blood path and negative pressure in the dialysate path causes excess H_2O to move from the patient (high pressure) to an area of lower pressure (the dialysate). The negative pressure is an actual suctioning force applied to the membrane.

PART

Endocrine System

··

⬭ **ADDISON'S DISEASE** (see also Aldosterone in Part 5, Renal System)

Addison's disease is due to hypofunction of the adrenal cortex of the kidney, causing a severe decrease in levels of aldosterone and cortisol with resultant fluid and electrolyte imbalances; protein, fat, and carbohydrate disturbances; and ultimately, circulatory collapse. Approximately 70% of the cases are idiopathic. Addison's disease is the "opposite" of Cushing's disease, in which there is an oversecretion of glucocorticoid hormones.

The pituitary gland secretes ACTH, which stimulates the adrenal cortex to secrete its own hormones. Addison's disease is diagnosed by stimulating ACTH with drug therapy and evaluating the response of the adrenal cortex. Normally, there is an increase in the excretion of hydroxycorticoids and ketosteroids, whereas patients with Addison's disease show little or no increase. Also, eosinophils in the patient's blood are measured. A drop of 60% to 90% in the count after ACTH is given is normal, but there is little drop in the count in a patient with Addison's disease.

(continued)

NOTES

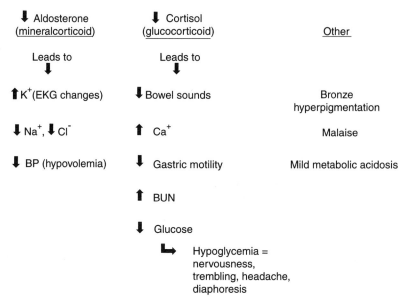

↓ Aldosterone (mineralcorticoid)	↓ Cortisol (glucocorticoid)	Other
Leads to ↓	Leads to ↓	
↑ K⁺(EKG changes)	↓ Bowel sounds	Bronze hyperpigmentation
↓ Na⁺, ↓ Cl⁻	↑ Ca⁺	Malaise
↓ BP (hypovolemia)	↓ Gastric motility	Mild metabolic acidosis
	↑ BUN	
	↓ Glucose	
	↳ Hypoglycemia = nervousness, trembling, headache, diaphoresis	

Figure 6-1 Signs and symptoms of Addison's disease. (Reprinted with permission. Jacobs, S.W. [1965]. *Structure and function in man.* Philadelphia: W.B. Saunders.)

Addisonian crisis is a life-threatening exacerbation of the disease with severe hypotension, shock, coma, and vasomotor collapse.

Treatment is based on fluid replacement with D5NS and the IV administration of corticosteroids.

REMEMBER: **No patient with Addison's disease should ever receive insulin. He may die from the resultant hypoglycemia.**

ADRENAL INSUFFICIENCY (see Addison's Disease, Cushing's Disease)

CUSHING'S DISEASE

Cushing's disease results from an oversecretion of ACTH by a pituitary or adrenal basophilic tumor, which in turn causes increased secretion of glucocorticoid hormones. It is diagnosed by the presence of high glucocorticoid metabolites in urine and plasma, indicating that adrenal hyperactivity exists. It is the "opposite" of Addison's disease, in which there is a severe decrease in the levels of aldosterone and cortisol.

(*continued*)

Signs and Symptoms

- Persistent hyperglycemia
- Protein tissue wasting (weakness, osteoporosis)
- K^+ depletion (dysrhythmias, renal disorders)
- Na^+ and H_2O retention (edema, hypertension, CHF)
- Abnormal fat distribution (moon face; buffalo hump; striae on breasts, axilla, legs)
- Increased susceptibility to infection
- Mood swings

The disease is treated by surgical removal of the causative tumor; drugs only are palliative for inoperative cancer.

DIABETIC KETOACIDOSIS (see also Hyperglycemic Hyperosmolar Nonketotic Coma)

Diabetic ketoacidosis (DKA) occurs when there is insufficient insulin to metabolize glucose.

(*continued*)

NOTES

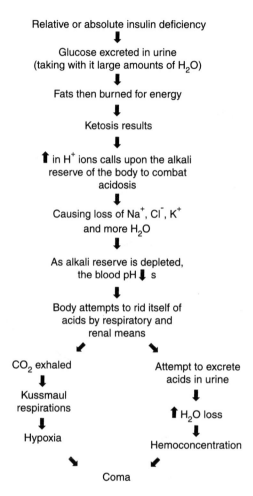

FIGURE 6-2 Diabetic ketoacidosis (DKA).

Signs and Symptoms

The signs and symptoms of DKA can be directly linked to three things:

1. Severe dehydration resulting in dry mucous membranes, thirst, loss of skin turgor, and an increase in serum osmolarity.

2. Loss of essential electrolytes resulting in a glucose >250 mg/dL (usually in the 600s).

3. Acidosis resulting in Kussmaul's respirations, acetone breath, and a positive anion gap.

(*continued*)

Therapy

The goal is to resolve the acidosis by stopping the breakdown of fats into ketoacids. The patient is usually placed on an insulin drip and maintained on same until the acidosis is resolved, the pH normalizes, and HCO_3 is >18 mEq/L. The glucose level may be within normal limits, but the former parameters must also be met before IV therapy can be discontinued and insulin changed to the SQ route. Initially, NS is given for volume restoration, followed with maintenance of ½ NS with KCl. Once the glucose level is below 250 mg/dL, IVs are changed to D5W or ½ NS with KCl.

REMEMBER: **Watch for the Somogyi effect (a paradox) whereby insulin causes a high blood glucose.** The rebound hyperglycemia is caused by the release of stress hormones to the insulin-induced hypoglycemia.

TABLE 6-1. Comparison of Hyperglycemic Hyperosmolar Nonketotic Coma and Diabetic Ketoacidosis

Hyperglycemic Coma	Diabetic Ketoacidosis
Patient with Type II diabetes and may be treated by diet alone, diet and an oral hypoglycemic agent, or diet and insulin therapy	Patient with Type I, insulin-dependent diabetes
Patient usually more than 40 years of age	Patient usually less than 40 years of age
Insidious onset	Usually rapid onset
Symptoms include	Symptoms include
1. Slight drowsiness, insidious stupor, or frequent coma	1. Drowsiness, stupor, coma
2. Polyuria for 2 d to 2 wk before clinical presentation	2. Polyuria for 1–3 d prior to clinical presentation
3. Absence of hyperventilation, no breath odor	3. Hyperventilation with possible Kussmaul's respiration pattern, "fruity" breath odor
4. Extreme volume depletion (dehydration, hypovolemia)	4. Extreme volume depletion (dehydration, hypovolemia)
5. Serum glucose 600 to 2,400 mg/dL	5. Serum glucose 300 to 1,000 mg/dL
6. Occasional gastrointestinal symptoms	6. Abdominal pain, nausea, vomiting, and diarrhea
7. Hypernatremia	7. Mild hyponatremia
8. Failure of thirst mechanism, leading to inadequate water ingestion	8. Polydipsia for 1–3 d
9. High serum osmolality with minimal CNS symptoms (disorientation, focal seizures)	9. High serum osmolality

(continued)

TABLE 6-1. Comparison of Hyperglycemic Hyperosmolar Nonketotic Coma and Diabetic Ketoacidosis (Continued)

Hyperglycemic Coma	Diabetic Ketoacidosis
10. Impaired renal function	10. Impaired renal function
11. HCO_3 level greater than 16 mEq/L	11. HCO_3 level less than 10 mEq/L
12. CO_2 level normal	12. CO_2 level less than 10 mEq/L
13. Anion gap less than 7 mEq/L	13. Anion gap greater than 7 mEq/L
14. Usually normal serum potassium	14. Extreme hypokalemia
15. Ketonemia absent	15. Ketonemia present
16. Lack of acidosis	16. Moderate to severe acidosis
17. High mortality rate	17. High recovery rate

DIABETES INSIPIDUS (see also Syndrome of Inappropriate Antidiuretic Hormone)

Diabetes insipidus (DI) is a disorder caused by a deficiency of the antidiuretic hormone (ADH) causing water **not** to be reabsorbed by the kidney tubules and resulting in excretion of large amounts of dilute urine. The disorder may appear slowly or develop suddenly, related to injury or infectious disease.

The *causes* of DI fall into two categories:

1. Vasopressin deficiency: The pituitary gland itself is defective due to idiopathic causes such as pituitary tumors, infectious processes, vascular accidents, neurosurgery, and so on.

2. Nephrogenic: Due to an inherited defect, the kidney tubules are unable to absorb water.

Signs and Symptoms

No matter what the etiology, patients routinely exhibit the following signs and symptoms:

- Polydipsia and polyuria (may drink 5 to 40 liters per day and excrete the same 5 to 40 liters per day). Unless the patient drinks almost continuously, there is always the danger of dehydration and hypovolemic shock.
- Decreased urine osmolality.
- Decreased urine specific gravity (<1.005).
- Increased serum osmolality.
- Increased serum Na^+.

(*continued*)

TABLE 6-2. Guide to Remembering DI and SIADH

	Serum Osmolality (285–295)	Urine Osmolality (50–1200)	Na+ (135–145)	Specific Gravity (1.010–1.030)
DI "dehydrated"	↑	↓	↑	↓
SIADH "waterlogged"	↓	↑	↓	↑

To help memorize this chart: **REMEMBER** the pneumonic *SUNG* for the titles across the top. Then remember that DI is listed first down the left side (alphabetically) and the "I" in DI indicates an increase, so the first category (serum osmolality) is **up**. Then alternate up, down, up, down across the column. For SIADH, remember it is opposite of DI (in many ways) and thus the first column (Serum Osmolality) is **down**. Alternate down, up, down, up across the column. Once committed to memory, differentiating DI and SIADH is easy.

The treatment for DI is with replacement ADH therapy. Desmopressin acetate (DDAVP) is a synthetic ADH and is given IV on an emergent basis or as a nasal spray for long-term therapy.

Aqueous vasopressin (Pitressin), IV or SQ, is sometimes used for transient or severe DI. It is short acting and may cause angina or hypertension. Dehydration and electrolyte imbalances must also be attended to, and replacement IV therapy with hypotonic solutions (½ NS) are administered, often to match the urine output on an hour-to-hour basis.

○ **DKA (see Diabetic Ketoacidosis)**

○ **GRAVE'S DISEASE**

In Grave's disease, excessive quantities of thyroid hormone are released related to heightened sensitivity to adrenergic stimuli. This causes the patient literally to "speed up" all bodily processes. Diagnosis is by the basal metabolic rate determination test (BMRD), the protein-bound iodine test (PBI), serum T_3 and T_4 determinations, and I^{131} urine excretion test (requires a 24-hour sample).

The patient presents with diaphoresis, tachycardia, and heat intolerance. Emotions are usually adversely affected, for example, extreme fatigue then episodes of overactivity. There is a characteristic bulging of the eyes (exophthalmos), and there may be a goiter due to hyperplasia and hypertrophy of the thyroid cells.

Treatment is with antithyroid drugs (propylthiouracil, Methimazole) or radioiodine therapy. Occasionally, surgery is required if the patient is unresponsive to drugs, and a subtotal thyroidectomy (removal of ⅚ of the gland) is performed.

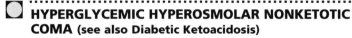

◉ HYPERGLYCEMIC HYPEROSMOLAR NONKETOTIC COMA (see also Diabetic Ketoacidosis)

Hyperglycemic hyperosmolar nonketotic coma (HHNK) is due to a relative (not total) insulin deficiency causing hyperosmolality of extracellular fluid and cellular dehydration. Enough insulin remains present to prevent ketone body formation. Etiology is related to mild diabetes, acute illness, trauma, diuretics, and steroids. Risk factors include pancreatitis, thiazide or steroid management, TPN or high-caloric feedings, and diet-controlled diabetes (see Table 6-1).

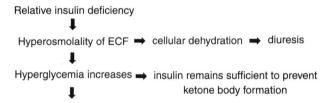

Relative insulin deficiency
↓
Hyperosmolality of ECF ➡ cellular dehydration ➡ diuresis
↓
Hyperglycemia increases ➡ insulin remains sufficient to prevent ketone body formation
↓
Osmotic gradient develops between brain and plasma
↓
Loss of brain H_2O
↓
CNS dysfunction (coma)

FIGURE 6-3 Evolution of HHNK.

Signs and Symptoms

- Serum glucose >650 mg/dL, usually >1,000 mg/dL
- Serum osmolality >350 mOsm/kg
- **Severe** dehydration (especially brain)
- No ketones
- No Kussmaul's respirations (shallow breathing only)
- No metabolic acidosis, normal anion gap

Treatment

Little, if any, insulin is needed. Main focus is replacing the volume deficit; patients may be depleted as much as 12 liters. The goal is to replace half of the fluid shortage in the first 24 hours. Normal saline, 2 or 3 liters over 2 hours, is initially started, and as vital signs recover, the patient is switched to ½ NS with KCl.

○ **HYPERTHYROID** (see Grave's Disease, Thyrotoxicosis)

○ **HYPOALDOSTERONISM** (see Aldosterone in Part 5, Renal System; Addison's Disease)

○ **HYPOPARATHYROID** (see also Hypocalcemia in Part 5, Renal System)

Hypoparathyroid is a clinical state resulting from the inadequate secretion of parathormone by the parathyroid gland, causing decreased levels of calcium and increased levels of phosphate. It is related to surgery of the thyroid gland, radiation injury to the thyroid, or pancreatitis.

Signs and Symptoms

These are related to a low calcium level (usually below 8.5 mg/dL) and an increased phosphate level:

- Numbness, tingling in fingers, toes
- Positive Chvostek's sign
- Positive Trousseau's sign
- Laryngeal stridor, dyspnea, cyanosis
- Confusion, seizures
- Prolonged QT on EKG

Treatment

The goal is to replete the calcium with supplements: 1 to 5 g orally TID, or 5 to 20 mL of a 10% IV solution at a rate not to exceed 0.5 mL/min. Do not mix in normal saline as it causes calcium excretion. Vitamin D supplements are given concomitantly to increase calcium absorption.

○ **HYPOTHYROID** (see Myxedema)

○ **MYXEDEMA** (Hypothyroidism)

Myxedema is a term used to describe a severe deficiency of the thyroid to secrete sufficient hormones to meet the requirements of the tissues that normally respond to the hormones. Lab tests such as T_3 and T_4, I^{131} uptake, and TSH are all decreased as evidenced by the patient exhibiting a slowing of all body activities (decreased metabolic rate and decrease of both physical and mental acuity).

(continued)

REMEMBER: "**Myxedema madness**" refers to the pronounced personality changes, such as paranoia and delusions.

There can be enlargement of the heart due to pericardial effusion and an increased tendency toward atherosclerosis and heart strain. Anemia may also be present along with a host of other symptoms ranging from cold, dry skin and weight gain to periorbital edema.

Treatment is based on thyroid hormone replacement with thyroxine, triiodothyronine, or combinations of these hormones.

PHEOCHROMOCYTOMA

A benign tumor of the adrenal medulla, pheochromocytoma causes increased secretion of epinephrine and norepinephrine resulting in proximal or sustained hypertension. It is often accompanied by severe headaches and the signs and symptoms of sympathetic activity are sweating, anxiety, palpitations, and so forth. The patient is at risk for CVA, cardiovascular damage, or sudden blindness. Severe symptoms can result in death.

Diagnosis

Diagnosis is made by the phentolamine (Regitine) test. After recording baseline blood pressure, an antipressor agent such as Regitine is administered IV. Blood pressure readings are taken at prescribed intervals until the pressure returns to its baseline level. A hypotensive effect lasting 10 to 15 minutes is diagnostic of pheochromocytoma, but a negative response does not rule it out.

Treatment

Treatment is surgical excision of the tumor. There is a high probability of profound shock 24 to 48 hours postop because catecholamine blood levels drop dramatically. There is also a high risk of hemorrhage because adrenal glands are highly vascular. The prognosis for removal of a benign tumor is good, however, and blood pressure usually returns to a normal level by the second or third postop day.

NOTES

PITUITARY GLAND: PHYSIOLOGY

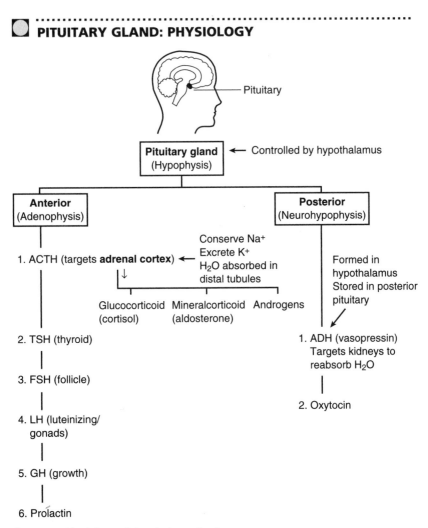

FIGURE 6-4 Physiology of the pituitary gland.

SYNDROME OF INAPPROPRIATE ANTIDIURETIC HORMONE

Syndrome of inappropriate antidiuretic hormone (SIADH) is a disease of the posterior pituitary characterized by sustained secretion of ADH, in spite of subnormal serum osmolality, resulting in water intoxication and hyponatremia. The patient is literally "waterlogged" (though edema

(continued)

may not be present). To positively diagnose SIADH, other causes of hyponatremia must be excluded, and renal, adrenal, and thyroid function must be normal (see Table 6-2).

Etiology

- Malignancy (especially oat cell cancer of the lung)
- Pulmonary disease
- Neurologic disorders (CVA, head trauma, etc)
- Hypothyroidism
- Drugs

Signs and Symptoms

A "syndrome" denotes a collection of symptoms, and therefore, the signs and symptoms can be subdivided according to origin.

TABLE 6-3. Origin of SIADH and the Associated Signs and Symptoms

Origin	Signs and Symptoms
Those due to **water intoxication**	Dilutional hyponatremia
	Decreased serum osmolality
	Increased urine osmolality
	Increased urine sodium
Those due to **hyponatremia** (dependent on severity and length of onset)	Fatigue, malaise
	Headache, confusion, neurologic damage
	Abdominal cramping
Those due to **other** causes	Weight gain without edema
	Increased urine osmolality
	Increased urine specific gravity
	Inappropriate urine Na$^+$ loss
	Increased circulating volume

The cornerstone of treatment is fluid restriction and is aimed at prevention of water intoxication and correction of electrolyte disturbances. Hypertonic saline, usually 3%, (see Hot Salt in Part 8, Drugs, Doses, Tables) and IV furosemide (Lasix) are given for an acute episode.

● THYROID STORM (see Thyrotoxicosis)

● THYROTOXICOSIS (see also Grave's Disease)

Thyrotoxicosis is a rapidly developing, life-threatening emergency characterized by greatly accentuated signs and symptoms of hyperthyroidism.

(continued)

Increased amounts of thyroid hormones are inappropriately released into the bloodstream, and metabolism is greatly exaggerated. Also known as "thyroid storm," it is a fatal event without intervention and is associated with a 10% mortality rate.

Signs and Symptoms

The signs and symptoms are related to the increase in the metabolic process:

- High fever, heat intolerance, diaphoresis
- Tachycardia (out of proportion to fever) with dysrhythmias (especially atrial)
- Tremors, muscle weakness
- Low TSH
- Elevated free T_4

Treatment

Treatment depends on the severity of the symptoms, but centers around suppressing hormonal release with iodides and giving propylthiouracil to block conversion of T_4 to T_3.

REMEMBER: **Always give propylthiouracil (PTU) at least 1 hour before the iodides.** Methimazole and propanolol (Inderal) may also be used, and plasmapheresis may ultimately be required.

REMEMBER: **Never give aspirin to these patients, as the drug increases the free T_3.**

Hematologic and Immune Systems

◻ AIDS

Acquired immune deficiency syndrome (AIDS) is an infectious disease caused by human T-cell lymphotrophic type III virus (HTLV-III). It is an acquired deficiency of the body's immune system. The immune system continually produces cells and antibodies that attack and destroy germs that otherwise would render a patient ill. The AIDS virus zeros in on certain T lymphocytes and breaks down the immunity, thus removing any natural resistance and leaving the patient vulnerable to a variety of viruses, bacteria, yeasts, fungi, and parasites. The virus is carried in the blood and transmitted through the blood.

Pneumonia is the major cause of death, usually due to the protozoa Pneumocystis or from the cytomegalovirus (CMV). The most characteristic cancer that develops is Kaposi's sarcoma. It spreads rapidly and is usually fatal. It may be initially limited to skin (red-brown lesions) but quickly spreads internally. Another cancer often developing is lymphoma, a cancer of the lymphatic system, which eventually causes death.

The screening tests for AIDS are (1) enzyme-linked immunosorbent assay (ELISA) test and (2) the Western blot test. Both look for antibodies produced by the immune system after infection by the virus and are therefore not accurate until a person has been infected for 4 to 12 weeks.

AIDS Profile

- Lymphocytopenia, thrombocytopenia
- Low $T_4 : T_8$ ratio
- Brain dementia (30% to 40%)
- Unexplained weight loss
- Night sweats
- Red-brown spots on skin or mucous membranes
- Swollen lymph nodes lasting more than 1 month
- Persistent white spots or unusual blemishes in the mouth

(*continued*)

- Fever >99°F for more than 10 days
- Persistent cough and shortness of breath
- Persistent diarrhea

Treatment

Treatment is with zidovudine (Retrovir) formerly called AZT. It decreases the replication of the AIDS virus but does not afford a cure.

ALBUMIN (see Transfusions)

ANEMIA

Hemolytic	Excessive erythrocyte destruction
Iron deficiency	Nutritional deficiency ($\downarrow$ MCV, $\downarrow$ MCH, $\downarrow$ MCHC)
Pernicious (aplastic)	Bone marrow failure resulting in decreased RBCs

NOTES

BLOOD, COMPOSITION OF (see also Body Fluid Compartments)

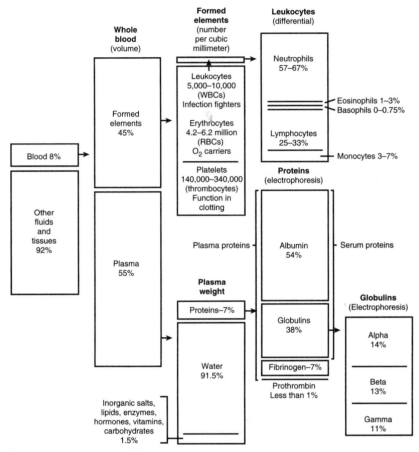

FIGURE 7-1 Composition of blood.

BLOOD PRODUCTS (see Transfusions)

NOTES

BODY FLUID COMPARTMENTS (see also Blood, Composition of)

Body fluid averages about 70% of total body weight, divided as follows:

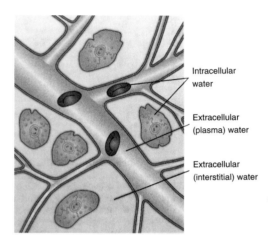

Intracellular water

Extracellular (plasma) water

Extracellular (interstitial) water

FIGURE 7-2 Distribution of body fluid. The extracellular space includes the vascular compartment and the interstitial spaces.

NOTES

⬤ CLOT FORMATION

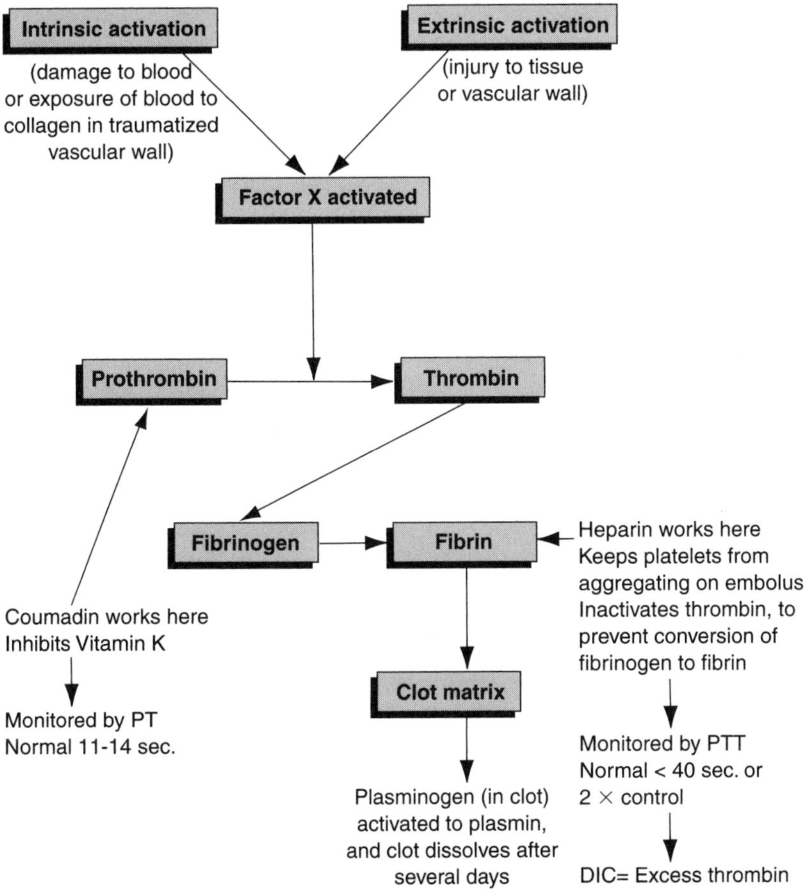

FIGURE 7-3 Clot formation. (Adapted from Bullock, B.L. [1996]. *Pathophysiology: Adaptations and alterations in function* [4th ed.]. Philadelphia: Lippincott-Raven.)

NOTES

● CLOTTING CASCADE

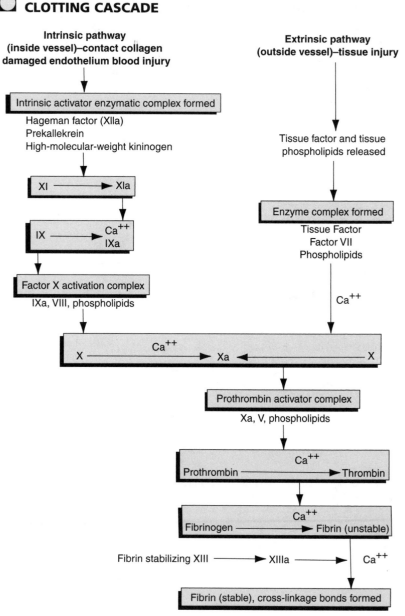

FIGURE 7-4 Blood coagulation sequence. a, Activated enzyme; Ca++, calcium is necessary in several reactions. Final common pathway begins with the activation of Factor X.

CLOTTING FACTORS

TABLE 7-1. Clotting Factors

Official Number	Synonym		Contemporary Version
I	Fibrinogen	I	(fibrinogen)
II	Prothrombin	II	(prothrombin)
III	Tissue thromboplastin	III	(tissue factor)
IV	Calcium	IV	(calcium)
V	Labile factor	V	(labile factor)
		VI	PF_3 (platelet coagulant activities)
		VI	PF_4
VII	Stable factor	VII	(stable factor)
VIII	Antihemophilic factor	VIII	AHF (antihemophilic factor)
		VIII	VWF (von Willebrand's factor)
		VIII	RAg (related antigen)
IX	Christmas factor	IX	(Christmas factor)
X	Stuart-Prower factor	X	(Stuart-Prower factor)
XI	Plasma thromboplastin (antecedent)	XI	(plasma thromboplastin antecedent)
XII	Hageman factor	XII	HF (Hageman factor)
		XII	PK (prekallikrein, Fletcher)
		XII	HMWK (high molecular weight kininogen)
XIII	Fibrin stabilizing factor	XIII	fibrin stabilizing factor

The Roman numerals and synonyms designating each clotting factor accepted by the International Committee on Blood Clotting Factors are located in the left-hand columns. Note the absence of factor VI. The version in the right-hand column incorporates more recently recognized clotting factors but is not officially recognized. (Green D. General considerations of coagulation proteins. *Ann Clin Lab Sci* 8[2]:95–105. Copyright 1987 by The Institute for Clinical Science, Inc. Reprinted with permission.)

CRYOPRECIPITATE (see Transfusions)

DEXTRAN (see Transfusions)

DISSEMINATED INTRAVASCULAR COAGULATION

Disseminated intravascular coagulation (DIC) is widespread hypercoagulation within arterioles and capillaries throughout the body. It is characterized by two opposing manifestations:

1. Diffuse fibrin deposition with resultant widespread clotting.

2. Hemorrhage from the kidneys, brain, adrenals, heart, and other organs.

(continued)

Etiology is unknown, possibly linked with thromboplastic substances entering blood (eg, metastatic cancer, OB complications, shock, sepsis, tissue damage from burns or trauma, snake bites, etc).

Pathophysiology

Release of thromboplastic substances
↓
Deposition of fibrin through microcirculation
↓
Microthrombi in brain, kidneys, heart
↓
Microinfarcts and tissue necrosis
↓
Red cells trapped in fibrin strands are destroyed (hemolysis)
↓
Platelets, prothrombin, and other clotting factors consumed in the process
↓
Free bleeding
↓
Excessive clotting activates fibrinolytic mechanism
↓
Production of fibrin split products
↓
Fibrin split products inhibit clotting function
↓
Further bleeding

NORMAL

arterio-venous shunt
open

Arteriole → → Venule

Capillary

Capillary perfusion is normal, blood flow is rapid.

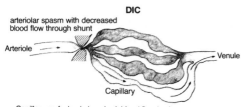

DIC

arteriolar spasm with decreased
blood flow through shunt

Arteriole → → Venule

Capillary

Capillary perfusion is impaired, blood flow is slow,
intracapillary thrombosis occurs with blood stagnation and acidosis.
Cells nourished by capillaries die of ischemia due to blood clotting.

FIGURE 7-5 Arteriole–capillary–venule relationship in normal circulation as opposed to the disseminated intravascular coagulation (DIC) patient. The effect of arteriovenous shunting in DIC is shown.

(continued)

Signs and Symptoms

- Prolonged PT/PTT, abnormal bleeding times
- Decreased platelets
- Increased fibrin split products
- Decreased fibrinogen (less circulating because used up in clot itself)
- Petechiae, ecchymosis in skin, mucous membranes, lungs (microhemorrhages)

Treatment

Treatment is centered on attention to the underlying cause. Heparin therapy is given to interrupt the clotting cycle and preserve clot factors. The use of blood products to replace loss is controversial.

⬤ FRESH FROZEN PLASMA (see Transfusions)

⬤ HESPAN (see Transfusions)

⬤ HODGKIN'S DISEASE

Hodgkin's disease is a chronic, progressive neoplastic disorder of unknown etiology characterized by enlargement of lymph glands, spleen, and liver. Proliferating cells are abnormal histocytes called Reed-Sternberg cells.

Staging:

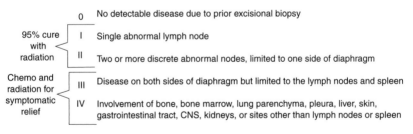

	0	No detectable disease due to prior excisional biopsy
95% cure with radiation	I	Single abnormal lymph node
	II	Two or more discrete abnormal nodes, limited to one side of diaphragm
Chemo and radiation for symptomatic relief	III	Disease on both sides of diaphragm but limited to the lymph nodes and spleen
	IV	Involvement of bone, bone marrow, lung parenchyma, pleura, liver, skin, gastrointestinal tract, CNS, kidneys, or sites other than lymph nodes or spleen

NOTES

⬭ LEUKEMIA

Leukemia is a group of malignancies caused by abnormal reproduction of white blood cells that create useless, immature cells called blasts. Blasts overpopulate bone marrow and spill into the bloodstream and lymph system. Patient has an elevated leukocyte count with a shift to the left.
There are *four types* of leukemia:

1. Chronic lymphocytic leukemia (CLL) (90% of leukemias)

   a. Gradual accumulation of abnormal lymphocytes

   b. Patient usually asymptomatic at diagnosis

   c. Disease of the elderly (>50 yr)

2. Chronic granulocytic leukemia (CGL)

   a. Accumulation and infiltration of myeloid cells

   b. 95% of cases show Philadelphia chromosome

   c. Seen in adults 25 to 60 years

3. Acute nonlymphoblastic leukemia (ANLL)

   a. Accumulation of immature myeloid leukocytes

   b. Seen in young adults to elderly >60 years

4. Acute lymphoblastic leukemia (ALL)

   a. Infiltration and accumulation of immature lymphoblasts

   b. Childhood leukemia in 80% to 85% of the cases

Treatment

Treatment is based on chemotherapy. For acute leukemia, the regimen includes three phases: induction (to achieve remission), consolidation (to further decrease cells), and maintenance (moderate doses over a prolonged time). For chronic leukemias, chemotherapy is usually oral, with minimal toxicity progressing to aggressive as the disease progresses. Sometimes radiation is used for lymph nodes or large masses. Bone marrow transplant, after old marrow has been ablated with chemotherapy and radiation, is an option providing a donor match can be found.

(continued)

NOTES

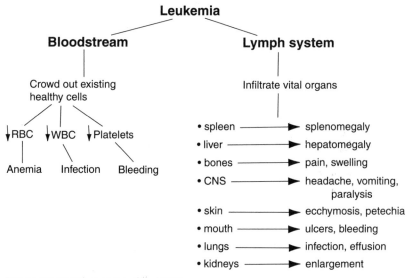

FIGURE 7-6 Manifestations of leukemia.

⬤ LYMPHOSARCOMA

Lymphosarcoma is a malignant condition of an unknown etiology, primarily involving lymphatic tissue. The earliest sign is **painless** enlarged lymph nodes. Eventually, lymphosarcoma invades bone marrow. The prognosis is poor, and treatment is palliative with radiation and chemotherapy.

⬤ MULTIPLE MYELOMA

Multiple myeloma is a neoplasm of the bone marrow that is rapidly fatal (from the Greek *myelo* marrow, *oma* tumor). The patient exhibits backache and bone pain; hyperglobulinemia; and a disruption of erythrocytes, leukocytes, and thrombocytes. The urine is positive for protein (Bence Jones). Treatment is palliative by amputating the affected bone.

⬤ PLASMA PROTEIN FRACTION (see Transfusions)

⬤ PLASMAPHERESIS (see Plasmapheresis in Part 1, Neurologic System)

⬤ PLATELETS (see Transfusions)

◯ RED BLOOD CELLS (see Transfusions)

◯ SHOCK, ANAPHYLACTIC

Anaphylactic shock is most commonly precipitated by antibiotic use (ie, iodine, penicillin). B lymphocytes secrete specific IgE antibodies in response to causative substance, resulting in a stimulation of mediator (ie, histamines) secretion. Histamine, in turn, causes systemic reactions: wheezing, laryngeal edema with bronchospasm, vasodilation, urticaria (macular eruptions on head and arms before spreading in a symmetrical pattern), and ultimately shock. The vasodilation causes increased capillary permeability, fluid loss resulting in hypovolemia, hypotension, and low cardiac output.

Epinephrine is the drug of choice for treatment (reverses bronchospasm, hypotension), along with diphenhydramine (Benadryl) (decreases the action of histamines). Albumin is given to draw fluid back into the intravascular space, and vasopressors are added to the regimen if needed (**no** Dobutamine).

◯ TRANSFUSIONS

Points to remember:

• Use only 0.9 NS for infusions. Lactated Ringer's solution causes agglutination, and dextrose causes hemolysis.

• Temperature of blood warmer should never be >98.6°F, or hemolysis can occur.

• After multiple units of blood, Ca^+ should be given to prevent hypocalcemia. (Do not mix Ca^+ in normal saline.)

• Transfusion reactions are of two types: nonhemolytic and hemolytic.
   The nonhemolytic type is the most common, usually seen in a patient receiving multiple transfusions. It is manifested by fever, chills, headache, a decreased BP, lumbar pain, and/or palpitations.
   The hemolytic type is more rare, usually related to the incompatibility of a blood group. The patient may have a very high fever, some times >104°F, with flushing, chills, lumbar pain, headache, chest pain, and/or dyspnea. He may progress to shock. Treatment is with fluids and diuretics.

(continued)

TABLE 7-2. Summary of Blood Compatability

% Pop.	Patient Type	Whole Blood	RBCs	FFP	Platelets	Cryoprecipitate
				Acceptable Donor Blood Types		
44	O	O	O	Any ABO type	Any ABO type	Any ABO type
43	A	A	A or O	A or AB	A or AB preferred	A or AB
9	B	B	B or O	B or AB	B or AB preferred	B or AB
4	AB	AB	Any ABO type	AB	AB preferred	AB
85	Rh$^+$	Rh$^+$ or Rh$^-$	Rh$^+$ or Rh$^-$	Rh$^+$ or Rh$^-$	Rh$^+$ or Rh$^-$	Rh$^+$ or Rh$^-$
15	Rh$^-$	Rh$^-$	Rh$^-$	Rh$^+$ or Rh$^-$	Rh$^-$ preferred	Rh$^+$ or Rh$^-$

ALBUMIN

Albumin is used as a blood volume expander in the treatment of hypovolemic shock, hemorrhage, trauma, acute hemodilution, or acute vasodilation. It improves "third space" fluid floss, including acute peritonitis, mediastinitis, burns, and postop radical surgery. It is used to reduce cerebral edema due to neurosurgery or anoxia. It is also used in the treatment of hypoproteinemia, hepatic cirrhosis, and nephrosis.

VOLUME:

5% (~ isotonic and isosmotic; 95% NS + 5% albumin)	250 to 500 cc bottles
25% (salt poor; 75% NS + 25% albumin)	50 cc (12.5 gm) or 100 cc (25 gm)

INFUSION RATE:

5%	1 to 10 cc/min; 25 to 60 minutes for 250 cc (more rapidly for patient in shock)
25%	Limit to no more than 4 cc/min; 12 to 25 minutes for 50 cc

(continued)

SPECIAL CONSIDERATIONS

No ABO blood group antibodies present; therefore, compatibility is not a factor.

CRYOPRECIPITATE

Cryoprecipitate is used to correct deficiencies of factor VIII (hemophilia A), von Willebrand's factor, factor XIII, and fibrinogen. It is occasionally used to control bleeding in uremic patients.

VOLUME:

Usually given as a pool of 10 to 20 units

INFUSION RATE:

1 to 2 mL/min (10 mL diluted component per minute)

SPECIAL CONSIDERATIONS:

Cryoprecipitate contains a small volume of plasma and no red blood cells. Plasma compatibility is preferred, but not required.

DEXTRAN 40

Dextran 40 is a hypertonic colloid solution that produces immediate and short-lived expansion of plasma volume (usually 1 to 2 times the Dextran 40 infused) by drawing fluid from the interstitial to the intravascular spaces. It is used in the treatment of shock due to hemorrhage, burns, surgery, or trauma.

VOLUME:

10% dextran 40 in 5% dextrose

10% dextran 40 in 0.9% NS

INFUSION RATE:

For shock, total dose during the first 24 hours should not exceed 20 mL/kg

Give the first 500 cc over 15 to 30 minutes; give repeated doses more slowly

Succeeding doses for a maximum of 4 additional days should not exceed 10 mL/kg

SPECIAL CONSIDERATIONS:

When stored for long periods, dextran flakes may form. To dissolve flakes, place container in warm water bath until solution clears.

Transient prolongation of normal bleeding time and coagulation profile may occur in high doses.

(continued)

DEXTRAN 70

Dextran 70 is a high-molecular-weight plasma volume expander with colloidal properties approximate to those of serum albumin. The expansion of the plasma volume is slightly in excess of the volume infused. It is used primarily for emergency treatment of hypovolemic shock or impending shock caused by hemorrhage, burns, and/or trauma. It is intended for use only when whole blood or blood products are not available, or when haste precludes the crossmatching of blood.

VOLUME:

500 cc

INFUSION RATE:

For emergency treatment of shock, the first 500 cc are given at 20 to 40 cc/min or over 13 to 25 minutes. In normovolemic patients, the flow rate should be no greater than 4 cc/min. Total daily dose should not exceed 20 mL/kg for the first 24 hours. If therapy continues beyond 24 hours, the total daily dose should not exceed 10 mL/kg.

SPECIAL CONSIDERATIONS:

The patient should be closely observed during the first few minutes of the infusion for evidence of an allergic reaction. Severe reactions have ended in fatalities.

Transient prolongation of normal bleeding time and coagulation profile may occur in high doses.

FRESH FROZEN PLASMA

Fresh frozen plasma (FFP) is used to increase the level of clotting factors in patients with a demonstrated deficiency. It is **not** used for volume expansion, as a nutritional supplement, or prophylactically with massive blood transfusions.

VOLUME:

200 to 250 cc (amount usually written on unit)

INFUSION RATE:

200 mL/hr or more slowly if circulatory overload is a potential problem

SPECIAL CONSIDERATIONS:

Plasma contains no red blood cells and crossmatching is not required; however, ABO-compatible plasma should be administered.

One unit should be thawed at a time because FFP must be used within 24 hours of thawing and using it later results in the loss of the labile clotting factors V and VIII.

Infuse using a blood filter or a component filter.

(continued)

HESPAN

Hespan (hydroxyethyl starch) is a synthetic colloid made from corn indicated for use as a plasma volume expanding agent in cases of shock from hemorrhage, trauma, sepsis, or burns. Expansion after infusion is equal to or greater than that produced by dextran 70 or 5% albumin.

VOLUME:

500 cc

INFUSION RATE:

Usual total dose is 20 mL/kg/day, but this is not an absolute

Total volume may be infused over 1 hour if the clinical situation demands

SPECIAL CONSIDERATIONS:

Serum amylase values can be approximately 2× normal after the Hespan infusion and is not indicative of pancreatitis.

Much lower risk of an allergic reaction than dextran.

May prolong coagulation profile and decrease platelets.

PLASMA PROTEIN FRACTION

PPF is a blood volume supporter used in the emergency treatment of hypovolemic shock due to burns, trauma, surgery, and infections. It is also used as a temporary measure in the treatment of blood loss when whole blood is not available. It is used to replenish plasma protein in patients with hypoproteinemia (if sodium restriction is not a problem).

VOLUME:

250 or 500 cc

INFUSION RATE:

Up to 15 mL/min, usual rate 1 to 10 mL/min

SPECIAL CONSIDERATIONS:

There are no ABO antibodies present, therefore compatibility is not a factor.

Hypotension can be associated with too rapid an infusion.

Similar to 5% albumin.

PLATELETS

Platelets are used to control or prevent bleeding associated with deficiencies in platelet number or function. They are used prophylactically for platelet counts <10,000 to 20,000. Do **not** transfuse platelets to patients with immune thrombocytopenic purpura (unless there is life-threatening bleeding) or use prophylactically with massive blood transfusions.

(continued)

VOLUME:

50 to 70 cc (one pack or unit represents the platelets removed from one unit of blood); usually given in "pools" of 6 to 10 units

INFUSION RATE:

Determined by volume tolerance, usually one pool over 10 minutes

SPECIAL CONSIDERATIONS:

Platelets are stored with gentle agitation at room temperature for a maximum of 5 days. Once bag is entered for pooling, platelets must be transfused within 4 hours.

Platelet concentrates contain few red blood cells; therefore, ABO compatibility is not required. Patients who are Rh⁻, however, generally receive Rh⁻ platelets. Under certain circumstances, it may be necessary to give these individuals Rh⁺ platelets.

Use a special component filter.

One unit of platelets should increase the platelet count by 6,000.

RED BLOOD CELLS (PACKED)

Packed red blood cells are used to increase the oxygen carrying capacity in anemic patients without a need for volume expansion. They are also used to replace acute or chronic blood loss. They are essentially whole blood with 80% of the plasma removed; they lack clotting factors and platelets.

VOLUME:

250 to 350 cc per unit

INFUSION RATE:

Depends on patient's volume status, usually 2 to 3 hours per unit (not to exceed 4 hours); more rapid if the clinical situation demands

SPECIAL CONSIDERATIONS:

Can cause the hemoglobin and hematocrit to rise faster than whole blood.

Hemoglobin up 1 g/dL and hematocrit up 2% to 3% per unit RBCs given.

Blood filter required.

WHOLE BLOOD

Whole blood is used to treat acute, massive blood loss requiring the oxygen-carrying properties of red blood cells along with the volume expansion provided by plasma. However, if the whole blood is >24 hours old, the platelets and clotting factors are no longer functional.

VOLUME:

400 to 500 cc blood plus 60 cc anticoagulant per unit

(continued)

INFUSION RATE:
As rapidly as necessary to stabilize the hemodynamic status

SPECIAL CONSIDERATIONS:
Acute blood loss of as much as one-third of a patient's total blood volume can often be managed with crystalloid and/or colloid solutions. Advances in the use of blood components have made whole blood transfusions rare; therefore, whole blood is not routinely used due to the excessive volume it affords.

24 hours may elapse before a rise in the hemoglobin and hematocrit can be seen.

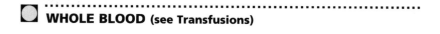

WHOLE BLOOD (see Transfusions)

PART

8

Drugs, Doses, Tables

⬤ **ADENOSINE**

Adenosine is a first-line antiarrhythmic used to treat PSVT and WPW. It has an unusually rapid onset and its half-life is less than 10 seconds.

- **Dose:** 6 mg IV rapid push over 1 to 3 seconds. After 1 to 2 minutes, if no resolution, give 12 mg IV rapid push over 1 to 3 seconds. May repeat one time in 1 to 2 minutes.

- **Precautions:** Immediately after administration, there is usually a distinct change in the EKG rhythm, such as PVCs, SB, or more commonly a short run of asystole. This usually resolves in seconds.

⬤ **ADRENALINE (see Epinephrine)**

⬤ **AMIKACIN (see Peaks and Troughs in Part 10, Labs)**

⬤ **AMINOPHYLLINE**

Aminophylline is a form of theophylline (aminophylline makes up 80% of theophylline) used to relax bronchial muscle spasm. It is used specifically for chronic and acute asthma, but it is sometimes employed for use in the patient with left ventricular failure and acute pulmonary edema (stimulating effect of the drug may increase cardiac output, while the decrease in pulmonary pressure relieves lung congestion and dyspnea).

- **For continuous IV infusion, mix:** 500 mg in 500 cc D5W or 0.9% NS.

- **Loading dose:** 6 mg/kg over 30 minutes (defer if serum theophylline level can be rapidly obtained).

- **Maintenance:** Up to 0.9 mg/kg/hr (usual dose 0.5 to 0.7 mg/kg/hr).

⬤ **AMPHOJEL (Aluminum Hydroxide)**

Amphojel contains no magnesium, but it decreases PO_4 levels by binding. It is used in renal patients.

⬛ AMRINONE (Inocor)

Amrinone is positively inotropic with vasodilator activity that decreases preload and afterload while increasing cardiac output. It is useful in short-term management of CHF.

- **Mix:** 500 mg in 100 cc 0.9% NS (never dilute with dextrose).

   REMEMBER: This adds 100 cc to the total volume in the bag.

- **Bolus:** 0.75 mg/kg over 2 to 3 minutes.

TABLE 8-1. Amrinone Initial Bolus

Weight (kg)	Infusion Rate (mL/hr)
40	6
45	7
50	8
55	8
60	9
65	10
70	11
75	11
80	12
85	13
90	14
95	14
100	15
105	16
110	17

- **Maintenance:** 5 to 10 μg/kg/min. If necessary, may administer another bolus after 30 minutes with an additional 0.75 mg/kg depending on response. Recommended dose is no greater than 10 mg/kg including bolus.

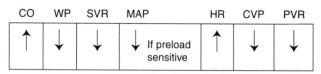

Figure 8-1 Amrinone at a glance.

(continued)

TABLE 8-2. Amrinone Maintenance

Dose (μg/kg/min)	5	6	7	8	9	10
Weight (kg)			Infusion Rate (mL/hr)			
40	5	6	7	8	9	10
45	5	6	8	9	10	11
50	6	7	8	10	11	12
55	7	8	9	11	12	13
60	7	9	10	12	13	14
65	8	9	11	12	14	16
70	8	10	12	13	15	17
75	9	11	13	14	16	18
80	10	12	13	15	17	19
85	10	12	14	16	18	20
90	11	13	15	17	19	22
95	11	14	16	18	21	23
100	12	14	17	19	22	24

- **Precautions:**
  - Precipitates with furosemide (Lasix).
  - May cause asymptomatic, reversible decrease in platelet count.
  - Alters liver enzymes.
  - Must be administered with caution if patient is allergic to sulfa.

BRETYLIUM (Bretylol)

Bretylium is an adrenergic blocking drug used in the treatment of ventricular fibrillation and ventricular tachycardia refractory to other therapy.

- **IV dose:** 5 to 10 mg/kg IV push over 8 to 10 minutes; may repeat in 15 to 30 minute intervals to a maximum total of 30 mg/kg in 24 hours.

  Alternately, a **continuous infusion** may be given:

- **Mix:** 2 g in 500 cc D5W.
- **Infuse:** 1 to 2 mg/min.

(continued)

NOTES

TABLE 8-3. Bretylium Maintenance

Dose (mg/min)	Infusion Rate (mL/hr)
1	15
2	30
3	45
4	60

- Precautions:
  - May cause severe hypotension.

○ **BREVIBLOC** (see Esmolol)

○ **CALAN** (see Verapamil)

○ **CARDENE** (see Nicardipine)

○ **CARDIZEM** (see Diltiazem)

○ **CEREBYX** (Fosphenytoin)

Cerebyx is indicated for short-term parenteral administration when other means of phenytoin administration are unavailable, inappropriate, or deemed less advantageous. It is used for control of generalized convulsive status epilepticus and prevention and treatment of seizures occurring during neurosurgery. *Cerebyx should always be prescribed in phenytoin sodium equivalent (PE) units.*

- **Dose:** Prior to IV administration, Cerebyx should be diluted in 5% dextrose or 0.9% NS for injection to a concentration ranging from 1.5 to 25 mg PE/mL.
- **Load:** 10 to 20 mg PE/kg given IV or IM. If administered IV, infuse at a rate no greater than 150 mg PE/min.
- **Maintenance:** 4 to 6 mg PE/kg/day.
- **Precautions:**
  - High risk of hypotension; be sure to administer IV slowly.
  - Observe patient throughout the period when maximal drug concentrations occur (10 to 20 minutes after completion of the infusion).

⬤ COUMADIN

Coumadin (warfarin) is an anticoagulant that inhibits vitamin K and directly interferes with clotting factors II, VII, IX, and X.

- **Dose:** 2 to 10 mg PO daily to maintain the PT at 1.5 to 2.5× control (ie, PT 21 to 35 seconds with control of 14 seconds).
- **Precautions:**
  - Anticoagulant effect can be reversed by 5 to 25 mg of vitamin K given IV.

⬤ DILTIAZEM (Cardizem)

Diltiazem is a calcium channel blocker used in SVT, atrial fibrillation, angina, and hypertension.

- **Dose:** 0.25 mg/kg IV push over 2 minutes (average 20 mg IV). If no response, may repeat in 15 minutes at 0.35 mg/kg over 2 minutes.
- **Mix:** 250 mg in 250 cc D5W
- **Infuse:** 10 to 15 mg/hr; titrate to heart rate.
- **Precautions:**
  - May cause bradycardia, headache, weakness, GI disturbances, dizziness.

⬤ DIPRIVAN (Propofol)

Diprivan is a premixed lipid emulsion that serves as a very short acting sedative and hypnotic. (It is **not** a paralytic.)

- **Infuse:** Begin with 5 μg/kg/min for a period of 5 minutes until onset of peak drug effect. When indicated, increase dose by increments of 5 to 10 μg/kg/min over 5- to 10-minute intervals. Usual maintenance dose is 5 to 50 μg/kg/min.

(continued)

NOTES

TABLE 8-4. Continuous Infusion Flow Rates (mL/hr) for Diprivan Maintenance

Dose (µg/min)	45	50	55	60	65	70	75	80	85	90	95	100	105	110	115	120	125	130
5	1	1.5	2	2	2	2	2	2	3	3	3	3	3	3	3.5	4	4	4
10	3	3	3	4	4	4	4.5	5	5	5	6	6	6	7	7	7	7.5	8
15	4	4.5	5	5	6	6	7	7	8	8	9	9	9.5	10	10	11	11	12
20	5	6	7	7	8	8	9	10	10	11	11	12	13	13	14	14	15	16
25	7	7.5	8	9	10	10.5	11	12	13	13.5	14	15	16	16.5	17	18	19	19.5
30	8	9	10	11	12	13	13.5	14	15	16	17	18	19	20	21	22	22.5	23
35	9.5	10.5	12	13	14	15	16	17	18	19	20	21	22	23	24	25	26	27
40	11	12	13	14	16	17	18	19	20	22	23	24	25	26	28	29	30	31
45	12	13.5	15	16	18	19	20	22	23	24	26	27	28	30	31	32	34	35
50	13.5	15	16.5	18	19.5	21	22.5	24	25.5	27	28.5	30	31.5	33	34.5	36	37.5	39
55	15	16.5	18	20	21.5	23	25	26	28	30	31	33	35	36	38	40	41	43
60	16	18	20	22	23	25	27	29	31	32	34	36	38	40	41	43	45	47
65	18	19.5	21.5	23	25	27	29	31	33	35	37	39	41	43	45	47	49	51
70	19	21	23	25	27	29	31.5	34	36	38	40	42	44	46	48	50	52.5	55
75	20	22.5	25	27	29	31.5	34	36	38	40.5	43	45	47	49.5	52	54	56	58.5

- **Precautions:**
  - Changes in rate should be made slowly (>5 minutes) to avoid hypotension and drug overdose.
  - Propofol causes a substantial decrease in BP in 25% to 40% of the patient population.
  - A specific line should be dedicated for administration. Solution is capable of rapid growth of multiple organisms.
  - Administration of bottle must be complete after 12 hours of spiking vial. Tubing and unused portion must be discarded at that time.
  - Tubing must be changed every 12 hours.

DOBUTAMINE (Dobutrex)

Dobutamine is a synthetic sympathomimetic catecholamine with inotropic, chronotropic, and vasodilator effects. It is useful in treating heart failure (especially with an increase in SVR and PVR) to increase contractility with no significant increase in heart rate. It is similar to dopamine but does not cause as significant a rise in blood pressure.

(continued)

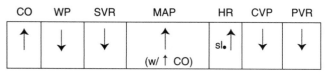

CO	WP	SVR	MAP	HR	CVP	PVR
↑	↓	↓	↑ (w/ ↑ CO)	sl. ↑	↓	↓

FIGURE 8-2 Dobutrex at a glance.

- **Infuse:** 2 to 10 μg/kg/min (can go up to 40 μg/kg/min with physician approval).
- **Mix:** 250 mg in 250 cc D5W or 0.9% NS.

$$\frac{16.67 \times cc/min}{weight\ (kg)} = \mu g/kg/min \qquad \textbf{or use Table 8-5}$$

TABLE 8-5. Doubtamine Maintenance (250 mg in 250 cc)

Dose (μg/kg/min)	2	3	4	5
Weight (kg)	Infusion Rate (mL/hr)			
50	6	9	12	15
55	6.5	10	13	16.5
60	7	10	14	18
65	8	11	16	19
70	8	12	17	21
75	9	13	18	22
80	9	14	20	24
85	10	15	21	25
90	11	16	22	27
95	11.5	17	23	29
100	12	18	24	30

- **Or mix:** 500 mg in 250 cc D5W or 0.9% NS.

$$\frac{33.33 \times cc/min}{weight\ (kg)} = \mu g/kg/min \qquad \textbf{or use Table 8-6}$$

(continued)

NOTES

TABLE 8-6. Dobutamine Maintenance (500 mg in 250 cc)

Dose (μg/kg/min)	2	3	4	5
Weight (kg)	Infusion Rate (mL/hr)			
50	3	4.5	6	7.5
55	3	5	6.5	8
60	4	5	7	9
65	4	6	8	10
70	4	6	8.5	10.5
75	4.5	6.5	9	11
80	5	7	10	12
85	5	7.5	10	13
90	5	8	11	13.5
95	6	8.5	11.5	14
100	6	9	12	15

DOPAMINE (Intropin)

Dopamine is a natural catecholamine that is the immediate precursor of norepinephrine. It is used to raise low blood pressure refractory to fluid therapy, to treat heart failure, to increase renal perfusion, and to correct hemodynamic imbalance in shock syndrome. Onset of the drug is rapid, usually 5 minutes, with a duration lasting about 10 minutes.

- **Infuse:**
  Low dose (renal perfusion): 1 to 3 μg/kg/min.
  Medium dose (increases contractility): 3 to 10 μg/kg/min.
  Medium dose (produces vasoconstriction): >10 μg/kg/min.
  High dose (works like Levophed): >20 μg/kg/min.

	CO	WP	SVR	MAP	HR	CVP	PVR
(<6 μg/kg/min)	↑	↑	sl. ↑	sl. ↑	↑	↑	↔
(>6 μg/kg/min)	↑	↑↑	↑↑	↑↑	↑	↑↑	↑

FIGURE 8-3 Dopamine at a glance.

(continued)

- **Mix:** 400 mg in 250 cc D5W or 0.9% NS.

$$\frac{26.67 \times cc/min}{weight\,(kg)} = \mu g/kg/min \qquad \text{or use Table 8-7}$$

TABLE 8-7. Dopamine Maintenance (400 mg in 250 cc)

Dose (μg/kg/min)	2	3	4	5
Weight (kg)	Infusion Rate (mL/hr)			
50	4	6	7.5	9
55	4	6	8	10
60	4.5	7	9	11
65	5	7	10	12
70	5	8	10.5	13
75	6	8	11	14
80	6	9	12	15
85	6	9.5	13	16
90	7	10	13.5	17
95	7	11	14	18
100	7.5	11	15	19

- **Or mix:** 400 mg in 500 cc D5W or 0.9% NS.

$$\frac{13.25 \times cc/min}{weight\,(kg)} = \mu g/kg/min \qquad \text{or use Table 8-8}$$

TABLE 8-8. Dopamine Maintenance (400 mg in 500 cc)

Dose (μg/kg/min)	2	3	4	5
Weight (kg)	Infusion Rate (mL/hr)			
50	8	11	15	19
55	8	12	17	21
60	9	14	18	23
65	10	15	20	24
70	11	16	22	26
75	11	17	23	28
80	12	18	24	30
85	13	19	26	32
90	14	20	27	34
95	14	21	29	36

(continued)

▪ **Or mix:** 800 mg in 250 cc D5W or 0.9% NS.

$$\frac{53.33 \times cc/min}{weight\,(kg)} = \mu g/kg/min \qquad \textbf{or use Table 8-9}$$

TABLE 8-9. Dopamine Maintenance (800 mg in 250 cc)

Dose (μg/kg/min)	2	3	4	5
Weight (kg)	Infusion Rate (mL/hr)			
50	2	3	4	5
55	2	3	4	5
60	2	3	4.5	6
65	2	3.5	5	6
70	3	4	5	6.5
75	3	4	6	7
80	3	4.5	6	7.5
85	3	5	6	8
90	3	5	7	8.5
95	3.5	5	7	9
100	4	5.5	7.5	9

▪ **Precautions:**
  • Renal ischemia occurs at high doses.
  • Causes tissue sloughing if IV infiltrates (use phentolamine [Regitine]).

EPINEPHRINE (Adrenaline)

Epinephrine is a potent catecholamine used to increase cardiac output by increasing heart rate, resulting in an increase in cerebral and coronary blood flow and an increase in SVR.

It is a first-line drug for any pulseless rhythm. Give 1 mg IV push every 3 to 5 minutes.

CO	WP	SVR	MAP	HR	CVP	PVR
↑	↑	↑	↑	↑	↑	↑

Figure 8-4 Epinephrine at a glance.

(continued)

- **Mix:** 1 mg in 250 cc D5W or 0.9% NS.
- **Infuse:** Start at 1 μg/min and titrate up to 10 μg/min for effect.*

   $0.067 \times \text{rate} = \mu\text{g}/\text{min}$ **or use Table 8-10**

TABLE 8-10. Epinephrine Maintenance

Dose (μg/min)	Infusion Rate (mL/hr)
1	15
2	30
3	45
4	60
5	75
6	90
7	105
8	120
9	135
10	150

- **Precautions:**
  - Do not mix with $NaHCO_3$.
  - Causes tissue necrosis if IV infiltrates.

   *Note: May be ordered in **μg/kg/min**. Start at 0.01 μg/kg/min and titrate up to 0.2 μg/kg/min for effect.

ESMOLOL (Brevibloc)

A β-adrenergic blocker, esmolol is used to control SVT or hypertension. It has a very short half-life.

- **Mix:** 5 g (20 cc) in 500 cc D5W or 0.9% NS.
- **Load:** 500 μg/kg/min for *1 minute.*

   (continued)

NOTES

TABLE 8-11. Esmolol Load

Weight (kg)	Infusion Rate (mL/hr)
50	150
55	165
60	180
65	195
70	210
75	225
80	240
85	255
90	270
95	285
100	300
105	315
110	330

- **Following load:** Run maintenance infusion for *4 minutes* at 50 μg/kg/min.

TABLE 8-12. Esmolol Maintenance

Dose (μg/kg/min)	50	100	150	200	250	300
Weight (kg)			Infusion Rate (mL/hr)			
50	15	30	45	60	75	90
55	16.5	33	49.5	66	82.5	99
60	18	36	54	72	90	108
65	19.5	39	58.5	78	97.5	117
70	21	42	63	84	105	126
75	22.5	45	67.5	90	112.5	135
80	24	48	72	96	120	144
85	25.5	51	76.5	102	127.5	153
90	27	54	81	108	135	162
95	28.5	57	85.5	114	142.5	171
100	30	60	90	120	150	180
105	31.5	63	94.5	126	157.5	189
110	33	66	99	132	165	198

- **If therapeutic effect not observed:** Repeat loading dose for *1 minute.*
- **After second load:** Run maintenance infusion for 4 minutes, increasing to 100 μg/kg/min.

(*continued*)

- **Continue** titrating, repeating loading infusion over 1 minute and increasing maintenance infusion in increments of 50 $\mu g/kg/min$ and running for 4 minutes.
- **End point:** When desired effect is reached, omit loading infusion and reduce incremental dose in maintenance infusion from 50 $\mu g/kg/min$ to 25 $\mu g/kg/min$ or lower. Usual maintenance dose is 50 to 300 $\mu g/kg/min$. Doses >200 $\mu g/kg/min$ do not significantly increase benefits.

FOSPHENYTOIN (see Cerebyx)

GENTAMICIN (see Peaks and Troughs in Part 10, Labs)

HEPARIN

Heparin inhibits the conversion of prothrombin to thrombin and prevents aggregation of platelets.

- **Mix:** 20,000 units in 500 cc D5W or 0.9% NS.*
- **Infuse:** Heparin dose should be titrated to keep the PTT 1.5 to 2× the pretreatment level. Normally the PTT is 30 to 40 seconds; accordingly, the treatment goal would then be a PTT of 60 to 80 seconds.

TABLE 8-13. Heparin (20,000 units in 500 cc)

Units hr.	cc's	Units hr.	cc's	Units hr.	cc's	Units hr.	cc's
40	1	720	18	1400	35	2080	52
80	2	760	19	1440	36	2120	53
120	3	800	20	1480	37	2160	54
160	4	840	21	1520	38	2200	55
200	5	880	22	1560	39	2240	56
240	6	920	23	1600	40	2280	57
280	7	960	24	1640	41	2320	58
320	8	1000	25	1680	42	2360	59
360	9	1040	26	1720	43	2400	60
400	10	1080	27	1760	44	2440	61
440	11	1120	28	1800	45	2480	62
480	12	1160	29	1840	46	2520	63
520	13	1200	30	1880	47	2560	64
560	14	1240	31	1920	48	2600	65
600	15	1280	32	1960	49	2640	66
640	16	1320	33	2000	50	2680	67
680	17	1360	34	2040	51	2720	68

Institution-specific.

⬤ HOT SALT

Hot salt is sometimes given to correct hyponatremia.

- One liter 3% NaCl contains 513 mEq sodium (500 cc = 256.5 mEq).
- 500 cc 3% NaCl is available as a premixed bag; 500 cc = 3 g NaCl.
- One 3% salt tablet = 1 g NaCl.

⬤ INOCOR (see Amrinone)

⬤ INSULIN

REMEMBER: If giving two types of insulin, draw up **clear first, then cloudy.**

REMEMBER: Regular insulin is the only type that can be given IV.

TABLE 8-14. Insulin

Action	Type	Onset	Peak	Duration	Hypoglycemia Most Apt to Occur
RAPID	Regular, SQ (crystalline zinc)	30–60 min	2–3 h	5–8 h	
	Regular, IV (crystalline zinc)	10–30 min	15–30 min	30–60 min	Before lunch
	Semilente	30–60 min	5–7 h	12–16 h	
INTERMEDIATE	Globin	2 h	8–16 h	24 h	
	NPH	60–90 min	8–12 h	24 h	Afternoon
	Lente	60–90 min	8–12 h	24 h	
SLOW	Protamine zinc	4–8 h	14–20 h	36 h	
	Ultralente	4–8 h	16–18 h	36 h	During night

⬤ INTROPIN (see Dopamine)

⬤ ISOPROTERENOL (see Isuprel)

⬤ ISUPREL (Isoproterenol)

Isoproterenol is a synthetic sympathomimetic agent with potent inotropic and chronotropic activity. It is used to increase the cardiac output by increasing the heart rate. It is no longer used in cardiac arrest.

- **Mix:** 1 mg in 250 cc D5W.
- **Infuse:** Start titration at 2 μg/min; may titrate up to 20 μg/min.

$$0.067 \times \text{rate} = \mu\text{g/min} \quad \text{or use Table 8-15}$$

TABLE 8-15. Isuprel Maintenance

Dose (μg/min)	Infusion Rate mL/hr
1	15
2	30
3	45
4	60
5	75
6	90
7	105
8	120
9	135
10	150
11	165
12	180
13	195
14	210
15	225
16	240
17	255
18	270
19	285
20	300

- **Precautions:**
  - Watch for tachycardia, ventricular irritability, chest pain.
  - Don't use any solution that is discolored.

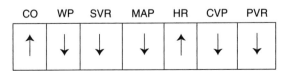

CO	WP	SVR	MAP	HR	CVP	PVR
↑	↓	↓	↓	↑	↓	↓

FIGURE 8-5 Isuprel at a glance.

◑ LABETALOL (Normodyne)

Labetalol is a β-adrenergic blocker used to control blood pressure in severe hypertension. It can be administered by either of two methods:

- **Repeated IV injection:** Give an initial dose of 20 mg IV slowly over 2 minutes. (This corresponds to 0.25 mg/kg for an 80 kg patient.) Additional doses of 40–80 mg can be given at 10 minute intervals, until the desired blood pressure has been reached or a total of 300 mg has been given. Maximum effect usually occurs within 5 minutes of injection.

- **Slow continuous IV infusion:** Mix 200 mg (40 cc) in 160 cc of D5W or 0.9% NS (to make a 1 mg/1 mL solution) and infuse at a rate of 2 mL/min to deliver 2 mg/min.

    Alternately, the drip can be mixed by adding 200 mg (40 cc) to 250 cc D5W or 0.9% NS (to make a 2 mg/3 mL solution) and infused at a rate of 3 mL/min to deliver approximately 2 mg/min.

- **Precautions:**
    • Because the half life of the drug is 5–8 hours, continuous IV infusion should continue only until the desired blood pressure is reached, at which time the patient should be started on a scheduled oral dosage regimen of the drug.
    • The patient should remain supine during administration, because a substantial decrease in blood pressure is expected.

NOTES

⬤ LEVOPHED (Norepinephrine)

Norepinephrine is a naturally occurring catecholamine that increases contractility and thereby increases blood pressure with only a mild increase in cardiac output. It is used to treat hypotension and a decreased SVR and to temporarily maintain organ perfusion. It causes an increase in myocardial oxygen consumption and myocardial ischemia.

- **Mix:** 4 mg in 500 cc D5W (8 μg/mL). Avoid dilution in 0.9% NS alone. Dependent on patient's fluid status, drip may need to be double concentrated to 4 mg in 250 cc (16 μg/mL) or quadrupled to 8 mg in 250 cc (32 μg/mL). To calculate the μg/mL infusion, use this formula:

$$\mu g/cc \times rate \div 60$$

- **Infuse:** Start at 0.5 μg/min and titrate to effect. Normal range is 2 to 12 μg/min; maximum is 30 μg/min. Therapeutic range varies widely from patient to patient.

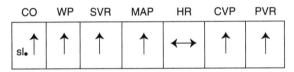

CO	WP	SVR	MAP	HR	CVP	PVR
sl.↑	↑	↑	↑	↔	↑	↑

FIGURE 8-6 Levophed at a glance.

NOTES

⬤ LIDOCAINE (see also Tocainide)

Lidocaine is an antiarrhythmic used to suppress ventricular irritability. It decreases automaticity and elevates the ventricular fibrillation threshold.

Lidocaine is a first-line drug for ventricular fibrillation or pulseless ventricular tachycardia. Give 1 to 1.5 mg/kg IV push. May repeat in 3 to 5 minutes up to total of 3 mg/kg.

- **Mix:** 2 gm in 500 cc D5W.
- **Infuse:** 1 to 4 mg/min.

TABLE 8-16. Lidocaine Maintenance

Dose (mg/min)	Infusion Rate (mL/hr)
1	15
2	30
3	45
4	60

- **Precautions:**
    - Drug can precipitate asystole or PEA.
    - Half-life increases after 24 to 48 hours of infusion; therefore, dose should be decreased after 24 hours and lidocaine levels monitored for toxicity.
    - Dose should be cut in half initially for patients with decreased hepatic blood flow.
- **For IV site discomfort** (institution specific): 100 mg to 1 L fluid.

⬤ MAALOX, MYLANTA (Magnesium Hydroxide)

Antacids that contain magnesium should not be used for renal patients.

⬤ MAGNESIUM SULFATE

Magnesium sulfate is used as a magnesium replenisher. It is also used to reduce the incidence of postinfarct arrhythmias.

- **For arrest status, torsades:** 1 to 2 g in 10 cc D5W IV push over 1 to 2 minutes.
- **As a replenisher:**
    Mix: 1 to 5 g in a 10% or 20% solution.
    Infuse: No faster than 1.5 mL/min of a 10% solution or 0.75 mL/min for a 20% solution.

● MILRINONE (Primacor)

Milrinone is an inotropic vasodilating agent with little chronotropic activity. It increases cardiac output without increasing myocardial oxygen demand or heart rate, and it decreases wedge pressure and vascular resistance. If patient is starting to require more dopamine and dobutamine, it may be time for this drug. It is used for short-term IV therapy of congestive heart failure or for calcium antagonist intoxication.

- **Mix:** 20 mg in 100 mL 0.9% NS or D5W (0.2 mg/mL).

- **Load:** 50 μg/kg administered over 10 minutes; response should be seen in 5 to 15 minutes. Patient "pinks up" and begins to diurese.

- **Infuse:** Dose titrated to hemodynamic and clinical response from 0.3 μg/kg/min to maximum of 0.75 μg/kg/min (0.5 μg/kg/min works well for 90% of patients).

TABLE 8-17. Milrinone Maintenance

Dose (μg/kg/min)	0.375	0.50	0.75
Weight (kg)	Infusion Rate (mL/hr)		
40	4.5	6.0	9.0
45	5.0	6.7	10.1
50	5.6	7.5	11.2
55	6.1	8.2	12.3
60	6.7	9.0	13.5
65	7.3	9.7	14.6
70	7.8	10.5	15.7
75	8.4	11.2	16.8
80	9.0	12.0	18.0
85	9.5	12.7	19.1
90	10.1	13.5	20.2
95	10.6	14.2	21.3
100	11.2	15.0	22.5
105	11.8	15.7	23.6
110	12.3	16.5	24.7

- **Precautions:**
  - Incompatible with furosemide and procainamide.
  - Hypotension should respond to IV fluids and Trendelenburg's position; use of vasopressors may be required.

NOTES

....
NEO-SYNEPHRINE (Phenylephrine)

Phenylephrine is a sympathomimetic adrenergic agent that acts by constricting the patient's blood vessels and raising the systolic pressure. This, in turn, stimulates baroreceptors in the carotid sinus and sets off reflex activity that slows the heart by increasing vagal tone. Phenylephrine resembles epinephrine with a more prolonged action and less effect on the heart.

- **Mix:** 20 mg in 250 cc D5W or 0.9% NS.
- **Infuse:** (To raise blood pressure rapidly) 100 to 180 μg/min.
- **Maintenance:** (When blood pressure stabilized) 20 to 80 μg/min.

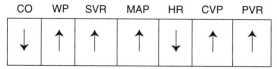

CO	WP	SVR	MAP	HR	CVP	PVR
↓	↑	↑	↑	↓	↑	↑

FIGURE 8-7 Neo-Synephrine at a glance.

 ....
NICARDIPINE (Cardene)

Nicardipine is a calcium channel blocker and potent vasodilator used for chronic stable angina and management of essential hypertension.

- **Mix:** 25 mg (10 cc) in 250 cc D5W or 0.9% NS (to make a 0.1 mg/mL solution).
  Do not mix with lactated Ringer's solution; not compatible with NaHCO$_3$.
- **Infuse:** Initially begin with 5 mg/hr (50 mL/hr) and increase by 2.5 mg/hr (25 mL/hr) every 15 minutes to a maximum of 15 mg/hr (150 mL/hr).
- **Precautions:**
  - Monitor closely for orthostasis and bradycardia.
  - If used concomitantly with digitalis, may increase digitalis level.

 ....
NIMBEX (Cisatracurium)

Cisatracurium (Nimbex) is a neuromuscular blocking agent used to ease endotracheal intubation or relax skeletal muscle during mechanical ventilation.

(continued)

NOTES

- **Mix:** Withdraw and discard 70 cc from a 250 cc bag of D5W or 0.9% NS (do not use lactated Ringer's solution).
  Add one 20-mL vial Nimbex (10 mg/mL) to bag.
  Concentration is 200 mg per 200 cc or 1 mg/mL.
- **Infuse:** 0.5 μg/kg/min to 10.2 μg/kg/min (average 3 μg/kg/min).

TABLE 8-18. Nimbex Maintenance

Dose (μg/kg/min)	1	2	3	4	5	6
Weight (kg)			Infusion Rate (mL/hr)			
30	1.8	3.6	5.4	7.2	9.0	10.8
40	2.4	4.8	7.2	9.6	12.0	14.4
50	3.0	6.0	9.0	12.0	15.0	18.0
60	3.6	7.2	10.8	14.4	18.0	21.6
70	4.2	8.4	12.6	16.8	21.0	25.2
80	4.8	9.6	14.4	19.2	24.0	28.8
90	5.4	10.8	16.2	21.6	27.0	32.4
100	6.0	12.0	18.0	24.0	30.0	36.0
110	6.6	13.2	19.8	26.4	33.0	39.6
120	7.2	14.4	21.6	28.8	36.0	43.2
130	7.8	15.6	23.4	31.2	39.0	46.8
140	8.4	16.8	25.2	33.6	42.0	50.4

- **Precautions:**
  - Nimbex does **not** provide pain relief.
  - Peripheral nerve stimulator should be used to monitor the neurologic response.
  - Onset is rapid (2 to 3 minutes) with peak effect in 3 to 5 minutes.
  - Recovery in 90% of the patients is within 25 to 93 minutes (half-life = 22 minutes).

NOTES

● NIPRIDE (Nitroprusside)

Nitroprusside is a venous and arterial dilator used to increase cardiac output by decreasing left ventricular afterload, to decrease blood pressure in hypertensive crisis, and to decrease pulmonary hypertension.

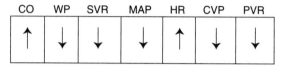

CO	WP	SVR	MAP	HR	CVP	PVR
↑	↓	↓	↓	↑	↓	↓

Figure 8-8 Nipride at a glance.

- **Infuse:** 0.5 to 10 μg/kg/min (usual dose is 3.0 μg/kg/min).
- **Mix:** 50 mg in 250 cc D5W.

$$\frac{3.33 \times cc/min}{weight\ (kg)} = \mu g/kg/min \quad \textbf{or use Table 8-19}$$

TABLE 8-19. Nipride Maintenance (50 mg in 250 cc)

Dose (μg/kg/min)	2	3	4	5
Weight (kg)		Infusion Rate (mL/hr)		
50	30	44	60	74
55	32	50	66	82
60	36	54	72	90
65	40	58	78	98
70	42	62	84	104
75	44	68	90	112
80	48	72	96	120
85	50	76	102	128
90	54	80	108	134
95				
100				

- **Or mix:** 100 mg in 250 cc D5W.

$$\frac{6.66 \times cc/min}{weight\ (kg)} = \mu g/kg/min \quad \textbf{or use Table 8-20}$$

(continued)

NOTES

TABLE 8-20. Nipride Maintenance (100 mg in 250 cc)			
Dose (µg/kg/min)	2	3	4	5
Weight (kg)	Infusion Rate (mL/hr)			
50	15	22	30	37
55	16	25	33	41
60	18	27	36	45
65	20	29	39	49
70	21	31	42	52
75	22	34	45	56
80	24	36	48	60
85	25	38	51	64
90	27	40	54	67

- **Precautions:**
  - Solution is stable for 24 hours only.
  - Cover IV bag with opaque shield; solution should not be exposed to light.
  - Check thiocyanate level if infusion continues longer than 72 hours or if rate ≥4 µg/kg/min.

NITROGLYCERIN (Tridil)

Nitroglycerin is a venous vasodilator used to decrease preload and afterload in left ventricular failure. It is also used for myocardial ischemia and as a dilator for coronary vasculature.

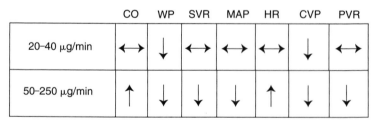

Figure 8-9 Nitroglycerine at a glance.

- **Infuse:** No optimum fixed dose; titrate to response. Usual rate is 5 to 20 µg/min, with increments of 5 µg/min every 3 to 5 minutes. (Sometimes ordered in µg/kg/min; usual dose is 0.1 to 5.0 µg/kg/min.)

(continued)

- **Mix:** 50 mg in 250 cc D5W.

$$3.33 \times \text{rate} = \mu g/\text{min}$$ **or use Table 8-21**

TABLE 8-21. Nitroglycerin Maintenance (50 mg in 250 cc)

Dose (μg/min)	Infusion Rate (mL/hr)
10	3
20	6
30	9
40	12
50	15
60	18
70	21
80	24
90	27
100	30
110	33
120	36
130	39
140	42
150	45
160	48
170	51
180	54
190	57
200	60
210	63
220	66
230	69
240	72
250	75
260	78
270	81
280	84
290	87
300	90
310	93
320	96
330	99
340	102
350	105
360	108
370	111
380	114
390	117
400	120

(continued)

■ **Or mix:** 100 mg in 250 cc D5W

$$6.66 \times \text{rate} = \mu\text{g}/\text{min}$$ **or use Table 8-22**

TABLE 8-22. Nitroglycerin Maintenance (100 mg in 250 cc)	
Dose (μg/min)	**Infusion Rate (mL/hr)**
10	—
20	3
30	5
40	6
50	8
60	9
70	10
80	12
90	14
100	15
110	17
120	18
130	19
140	21
150	23
160	24
170	26
180	27
190	29
200	30
210	32
220	33
230	35
240	36
250	38
260	39
270	41
280	42
290	44
300	45
310	47
320	48
330	50
340	51
350	53
360	54
370	56
380	57
390	59
400	60

(*continued*)

- **Precautions:**
  - Comes premixed in a glass bottle; use special nonadsorbing tubing.
  - If piggybacking, do so close to insert site as tubing can adsorb 40% to 80% of the drug.
  - Solution stable only 24 hours.
  - Some patients develop a tolerance over 1 to 2 days.

○ **NITROPRUSSIDE (see Nipride)**

○ **NORCURON (see Vecuronium)**

○ **NOREPINEPHRINE (see Levophed)**

○ **NORMODYNE (see Labetalol)**

○ **PHENYLEPHRINE (see Neo-Synephrine)**

○ **PITRESSIN**

Pitressin, or synthetic ADH, is used in patients with diabetes insipidus to cause water reabsorption by the kidneys and also to provide vasoconstriction in patients with portal hypertensive bleeding.

- **Mix:** 100 units in 250 cc 0.9% NS.
- **Infuse:** 0.1 to 0.4 U/min.

TABLE 8-23. Pitressin Maintenance

Dose (U/min)	Infusion Rate (mL/hr)
0.1	6
0.2	12
0.3	18
0.4	24

- **Precautions:**
  - Doses up to 1.0 U/min are sometimes necessary to control bleeding, but this significantly increases the risk of toxicity.
  - Tapering down before discontinuation is not necessary.

◯ PRIMACOR (see Milrinone)

◯ PROCAINAMIDE (Pronestyl)

Procainamide is an antiarrhythmic and antifibrillatory drug used to treat ectopy and recurrent ventricular tachycardia refractory to lidocaine.

- **Emergency status:** Give 20 mg/min IV until dysrhythmia is suppressed, the QRS widens by 50%, there is hypotension, or a total of one gram has been given.
- **For infusion, mix:** 2 gm in 500 cc D5W.
- **Infuse:** 1 to 4 mg/min.

TABLE 8-24. Procainamide Maintenance

Dose (mg/min)	Infusion Rate (mL/hr)
1	15
2	30
3	45
4	60

- **Precautions:**
  - Check blood levels; effective procainamide concentrations are 4 to 8 μg/ml.
  - Levels >16 μg/mL are associated with toxicity (usually in renal patients or a high dose infusion for greater than 24 hours).

◯ PRONESTYL (see Procainamide)

◯ PROPOFOL (see Diprivan)

◯ THEOPHYLLINE (see Aminophylline)

◯ TOBRAMYCIN (see Peaks and Troughs in Part 10, Labs)

◯ TOCAINIDE (see also Lidocaine)

Tocainide is the oral analogue of lidocaine.

- **Initial dose:** 400 mg every 8 hours. Usual adult daily dose: 1200 to 1800 mg/day in 3 divided doses.

○ ......
TRIDIL (see Nitroglycerin)

○ ......
VANCOMYCIN (see Peaks and Troughs in Part 10, Labs)

○ ......
VECURONIUM (Norcuron)

Vecuronium is an intermediate-acting neuromuscular blockage agent usually used during surgery to provide skeletal muscle relaxation. Unlabeled use in the ICU setting as a continuous infusion to facilitate mechanical ventilation.

- **Mix:** 100 mg in 100 mL D5W or 0.9% NS.
- **Continuous infusion:** 0.5 to 2 μg/kg/min (0.8 to 1.2 μg/kg/min average range).
- Precautions
  - Vecuronium does **not** provide pain relief.
  - Peripheral nerve stimulator should be used to monitor neurologic response.
  - Continuous infusion raises the concern for drug-induced myopathies in the ICU setting.
  - Prolonged weakness persists in some patients after discontinuation of drug.
  - Solution should be discarded 24° after reconstitution.

○ ......
VERAPAMIL (Calan)

Verapamil is a calcium channel blocker that slows conduction and prolongs refractoriness in the AV node. It is used to slow the ventricular response in atrial fibrillation, atrial flutter, and PSVT.

- **Dose:** Give 2.5 to 5 mg IV push slowly over 2 minutes. If no response in 15 to 30 minutes, may give second dose of 5 to 10 mg IV push slowly over 2 to 4 minutes.
- **Precautions:**
  - **Never** give verapamil to a patient with wide complex PSVT (odds are 100:1 that if QRS is wide and rhythm is a ventricular tachycardia, patient will arrest if given verapamil).
  - Don't give within 30 minutes of IV propranolol (Inderal) because it may cause asystole.
  - Transient hypotension is expected.

9

Conversions, Calculations, Compatibility

⬤ CALCULATING DRUG DOSES

Here is the **easiest** way to figure out drip rate or μg/kg/min for any drip. Once you remember this formula, it is **all you need to know** to get you quickly through calculations. You're going to figure a **constant,** but you need to remember that *every time a drip concentration changes or the patient's weight changes, the constant changes.*

Here's how it works:

1. Divide the mg in the solution by the cc in the solution

2. Divide that by the patient's weight in kg

3. Divide that by 60 (min/hr)

4. Multiply the whole thing by 1000 (μg/mg)

5. The result of the first four steps yields your **constant**

6. Now, all you have to do is multiply your constant by the drip rate, and you have your μg/kg/min

REMEMBER: Every time the drip rate changes, you need to remultiply to get the correct μg/kg/min, but the constant remains the same as long as the drip concentration and the patient's weight remain the same.

For example:

800 mg dopamine in 500 cc D5W. Patient's weight is 70 kg.

Drip was hung in an emergency situation, and you arbitrarily started it at 13 mL/hr.

$$800 \div 500 \div 70 \div 60 \times 1000 = 0.380 \text{ (constant)}$$
$$13 \times 0.380 = 5 \ \mu\text{g/kg/min}$$

(continued)

Patient's status deteriorates. You raise the drip rate to 16 mL/hr. Because you already know the **constant,** you need only multiply it by the new drip rate:

$$16 \times 0.380 = 6 \ \mu g/kg/min$$

This formula can also work in reverse. **You know μg/kg/min but want the drip rate.**
For example:

100 mg nitroprusside (Nipride) in 250 cc D5W. Patient weight is 70 kg. Orders to start at 3 μg/kg/min.

Figure your constant:

$$100 \div 250 \div 70 \div 60 \times 1000 = 0.095 \ (\text{constant})$$

Now you "play" with it. Arbitrarily pick a drip rate to start, say 8.

$$8 \times 0.095 = 0.76 \ \mu g/kg/min$$

You know that's not enough (orders for 3 μg/kg/min), and a cursory estimate shows that four times your original rate would be a lot closer. (If 8 = 0.76, then 32 must equal somewhere about 2.8.)

$$32 \times 0.095 = 3.04 \ \mu g/kg/min$$

Almost perfect, but check to see if 31 would do it exactly:

$$31 \times 0.095 = 2.94 \ \mu g/kg/min$$

⬤ **ALTERNATE METHOD FOR CALCULATIONS**

• **Know IV Rate of Infusion (mL/hr); Want μg/kg/min**

$$\frac{\text{Unknown flow rate } (x) \times \text{weight (kg)} \times 60 \times \text{amount of fluid in bag (cc)}}{\text{amount of drug in bag converted to } \mu g} = \text{rate of infusion (mL/hr)}$$

Example:

Nipride (100 mg in 250 cc D5W) is infusing at 20 mL/hr. Patient weight is 65 kg.

$$\frac{\text{Unknown } (x) \times 65 \times 60 \times 250}{100,000} = 20 \ \text{mL/hr}$$
$$10x = 20 \ \text{mL/hr}$$
$$x = 2 \ \mu g/kg/min$$

(continued)

• Know µg/kg/min; Want IV Flow Rate (mL/hr)

$$\frac{\mu g/kg/min \times weight\ (kg) \times 60 \times amount\ of\ fluid\ in\ bag\ (cc)}{amount\ of\ drug\ in\ bag\ converted\ to\ \mu g} = y$$

Example:

500 mg dobutamine (Dobutrex) in 250 cc D5W. Orders to start drip at 3 µg/kg/min. Patient weight is 70 kg.

$$\frac{3 \times 70 \times 60 \times 250}{500,000} = 6\ mL/hr$$

• Know Units in Solution; Want IV Drip Rate in cc/hr

$$\frac{Units\ in\ solution}{cc's\ of\ solution} = units\ per\ cc$$

Example:

20,000 units heparin in 500 cc D5W. Ordered to infuse at 1200 U/hr. Set up equation:

$$\frac{20,000\ units}{500\ cc} = 40\ units\ per\ cc$$

Use the product of that equation (40 units/cc) to calculate the unknown:

40 units is to 1 cc

as

1200 units is to x

Cross multiply:

$$40x = 1200$$
$$x = 30\ cc/hr\ to\ be\ infused$$

NOTES

TABLE 9-1. Compatibility Chart

	Aminophylline	Amphotericin B	Ampicillin	Atropine	Calcium gluconate	Carbenicillin	Cefazolin	Cimetidine	Clindamycin	Diazepam	Dopamine	Epinephrine	Erythromycin	Fentanyl	Furosemide	Gentamicin
Aminophylline	•	Y		Y	N	N		N	Y	Y	N	N				
Amphotericin B		•	N		N	N		N			N					N
Ampicillin	Y	N	•	N	N	Y	Y		N		N		N			N
Atropine			N	•			Y			N		N		Y		
Calcium gluconate	Y	N	N		•		N		N		Y	N	Y			
Carbenicillin	N	N	Y			•	Y	Y			Y	N	N			N
Cefazolin	N		Y		N		•	N		Y			N			N
Cimetidine		N		Y		Y	N	•	Y			Y	Y	Y		
Clindamycin	N		N		N	Y		Y	•							Y
Diazepam	Y		N				Y			•		N			N	
Dopamine	Y	N	N		Y	Y					•					Y
Epinephrine	N			N	N	N		Y		N		•	N		N	
Erythromycin	N		N		Y	N	N	Y				N	•			
Fentanyl				Y										•		
Furosemide								Y		N		N			•	N
Gentamicin		N	N			N	N	Y	Y		N				N	•
Glycopyrrolate				Y							N					
Heparin sodium	Y	Y	Y	N	Y			Y	Y	N	Y	Y	N		Y	N
Hydrocortisone	Y	Y	N		Y	Y	Y		Y		Y		Y			
Hydroxyzine	N			Y						N				Y		
Levarterenol	N			N	Y	N	N	Y		N		N			N	
Lidocaine	Y	N	Y		Y	Y	N	Y		N	Y	N	Y			
Meperidine	N			Y						N		Y		Y		
Morphine	N			Y						N		Y		Y		
Nitroglycerin	Y											Y		Y		
Pentobarbital	Y			N				N	N	N				N	N	
Potassium chloride	Y	N	Y	Y	Y	Y	Y	Y	Y	N	Y	N	Y		Y	
Sodium bicarbonate	Y	Y		N	N				Y	N		N	Y			
Tetracycline	N	N	N			N	N	N	Y			Y			N	
Vancomycin	N			Y				Y					Y			
Verapamil	Y	N	Y	Y	Y	Y	Y	Y	Y	Y	Y	Y	Y		Y	Y
Vitamin B & C complex	N		Y	Y	Y	N	Y	Y	Y	N	Y	Y	N		Y	Y

Glycopyrrolate	Heparin sodium	Hydrocortisone	Hydroxyzine	Levarterenol	Lidocaine	Meperidine	Morphine	Nitroglycerin	Pentobarbital	Potassium chloride	Sodium bicarbonate	Tetracycline	Vancomycin	Verapamil	Vitamin B & C complex	
Y	Y	N	N	Y	N	N	Y	Y	Y	Y	N	N	Y		N	Aminophylline
Y	Y		N							N	Y	N		N		Amphotericin B
Y	N		Y							Y		N		Y	Y	Ampicillin
Y	N		Y	N		Y	Y		N	Y				Y	Y	Atropine
Y	Y		Y	Y						Y	N	N	Y	Y	Y	Calcium gluconate
	Y		N	Y						Y		N		Y	N	Carbenicillin
	Y		N	N				N		Y		N		Y	Y	Cefazolin
Y			Y	Y				N		Y		Y	Y	Y	Y	Cimetidine
Y	Y							N		Y	Y			Y	Y	Clindamycin
N	N		N	N	N	N	N		N	N	N			Y	N	Diazepam
Y	Y		Y		Y			Y		Y		Y	Y	Y	Y	Dopamine
Y			N	N	Y					N	N			Y	Y	Epinephrine
N	Y			Y				N	Y	Y	N	Y	Y	Y	N	Erythromycin
		Y			Y	Y		N						Y		Fentanyl
Y			N				Y			Y		N		Y	Y	Furosemide
N														Y	Y	Gentamicin
•		Y		Y	Y	Y		N		N						Glycopyrrolate
	•	N	N	Y	Y	N	N			Y	Y	N	N	Y	Y	Heparin sodium
Y	N	•	Y	Y				N	Y	Y	N	Y	Y	Y	Y	Hydrocortisone
Y	N	Y	•	Y	Y	Y			N						N	Hydroxyzine
Y	Y	Y	Y	•			Y	Y	Y	Y	Y		Y	Y	Y	Levarterenol
Y	Y	Y	Y		•		Y	Y	Y	Y	Y		Y	Y	Y	Lidocaine
Y	N	Y				•	N	N		Y			Y			Meperidine
Y	N	Y			N	N	•	N	Y	N			Y		Y	Morphine
		Y						•						Y		Nitroglycerin
N		N	N	N	Y	N	N		•		N	N	N	Y		Pentobarbital
Y	Y		Y	Y		Y				•	Y	Y	Y	Y	Y	Potassium chloride
N	Y	Y		Y	Y	N	N		N	Y	•	N	N	Y	N	Sodium bicarbonate
N	N			Y	Y			N	Y	N		•			Y	Tetracycline
N	Y							N	Y	N			•	Y	Y	Vancomycin
Y	Y		Y	Y	Y	Y	Y	Y	Y	Y	Y		Y	•	Y	Verapamil
Y	Y	N	Y	Y		Y				N	Y	Y	Y		•	Vitamin B & C complex

Key: Y = compatible; N = incompatible; blank space = information about compatibility was not available.

Note: Because the compatibility of two or more drugs in solution depends on several variables such as the solution itself, drug concentration, and the method of mixing (bottle, syringe, or Y-site), this table is intended to be used solely as a guide to general drug compatibilities. Before mixing any drugs, the health care professional should ascertain if a potential incompatibility exists by referring to an appropriate information source.

(Reprinted from Malseed R.T., Goldstein F.J., Balkon N. (1995) *Pharmacology: Drug Therapy and Nursing Management*, 4th ed. Philadelphia: JB Lippincott.)

● CONVERSION REFERENCES

Height

Height (inches) $\times$ 2.54 = height in cm (one inch = 2.54 cm)

TABLE 9-2. Height Conversion

Feet, Inches	cm
4, 10	147
4, 11	148
5, 0	152
5, 1	155
5, 2	157
5, 3	160
5, 4	162
5, 5	165
5, 6	167
5, 7	170
5, 8	172
5, 9	175
5, 10	178
5, 11	180
6, 0	182
6, 1	185
6, 2	188
6, 3	190
6, 4	193
6, 5	195
6, 6	198
6, 7	200
6, 8	203
6, 9	205
6, 10	208

(*continued*)

NOTES

Weight

Weight (lb) divided by 2.2 kg = weight in kg (1 lb = 0.453 kg)
Weight (kg) × 2.2 lb = weight in lb (1 kg = 2.2 lb)

TABLE 9-3. Weight Conversion

lb	kg
22	10
33	15
44	20
55	25
66	30
77	35
88	40
99	45
110	50
121	55
132	60
143	65
154	70
165	75
176	80
187	85
198	90
209	95
220	100
231	105
242	110
253	115
264	120
275	125

(continued)

N O T E S

Temperature

Fahrenheit $- 32 \times 0.555 =$ centigrade
Centigrade $\times 1.8 + 32 =$ Fahrenheit

TABLE 9-4. Temperature Conversion

°C	°F
40.6	105.1
40.4	104.7
40.2	104.3
40.0	104.0
39.8	103.7
39.6	103.3
39.4	102.9
39.2	102.6
39.0	102.2
38.8	101.8
38.6	101.5
38.4	101.2
38.2	100.8
38.0	100.4
37.8	100.1
37.6	99.7
37.4	99.3
37.2	99.0
37.0	*98.6*
36.0	96.8
35.0	95.0
34.0	93.2
33.0	91.4
32.0	89.6
31.0	87.8
30.0	86.0
29.0	85.2
28.0	82.4
27.0	80.6

NOTES

DOSAGE EQUIVALENTS

Weight

1 kg = 2.2 lb

1 lb = 454 grams

1 grain = 65 mg

60 grains = 1 dram

1 ounce = 30 gm

8 drams = 1 ounce

1/65 grain = 1 mg

15 grains = 1 gm

5 grains = 325 mg

Volume

1 tbsp = 15 cc

1 tsp = 5 cc

15 minims = 1 cc

1 quart = 946 cc

1 liter = 1000 cc

1 fl dram = 4 cc

1 fl oz = 30 cc

Length

1 inch = 2.54 cm

39.4 inch = 1 meter

1 km = 0.6 mile

1 cm = 0.4 inch

FIGURE 9-1 Dosage equivalents.

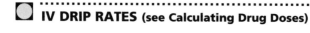

● **IV DRIP RATES (see Calculating Drug Doses)**

● **IV FLUID THERAPY (see also Body Fluid Compartments in Part 7, Hematologic and Immune Systems)**

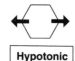

Hypotonic

Provides salt and H_2O. Moves fluid into cell to hydrate cell; results in intracellular expansion; decreases intravascular osmolality.

1/2 NS	77 mEq/L Na⁺
	77 mEq/L Cl⁻
	154 mOsm/L

.33% NS

2.5% Dextrose

D5W	Provides hydration

Isotonic

Provides hydration.
Maintains same osmotic pressure as blood; therefore, cellular components unchanged.

0.9% NS	154 mEq/L Na⁺
	154 mEq/L Cl⁻
	08 mOsm/L

LR	130 mEq/L Na⁺
	109 mEq/L Cl⁻
	4 mEq/L K⁺
	27 mEq/L lactate
	274 mOsm/L

D5W	Isotonic in bag only

Hypertonic

Replaces sodium.
Pulls fluid from cell and shifts into intravascular space, resulting in interstitial dehydration. Increases intravascular osmolality.

3% NS	512 mEq/L Na⁺
	513 mEq/L Cl⁻
	1026 mOsm /L

D5 1/2 NS	Provides Na⁺, Cl⁻
D5 1/4 NS	Provides Na⁺, Cl⁻
D5 NS	Provides fluid
D5 LR	Increases interstitial fluid pressure
D10 LR	Maintains volume (expander) Supplies blood lactate ions
D50 W	Increases blood sugar when given rapidly
D20 W	Provides calories in small amount of fluid
D10 W	Provides calories in small amount of fluid

FIGURE 9-2 IV fluids.

(continued)

REMEMBER:

• Never use lactated Ringer's solution if the patient is alkalotic (a normal liver converts the lactate to bicarbonate).

• Never use lactated Ringer's solution if the patient has liver disease (a diseased liver produces lactic acid and ammonia as by-products).

PART

10

Labs

☐ **DRUG LEVELS** (see Therapeutic Drug Levels)

☐ **DRUG PEAKS AND TROUGHS** (see Peaks and Troughs)

☐ **LAB FINDINGS SUGGESTIVE OF MEDICAL DISORDERS**

TABLE 10-1. Lab Findings, Electrolytes

Electrolytes

Ca^+ ↑ Acidosis, acute renal failure, bone metastases, carcinoma, adrenal hypofunction, hyperparathyroidism, hyperthyroidism
↓ Hypoparathyroidism, renal insufficiency, Cushing's syndrome, acute pancreatitis, ulcerative colitis

Cl^- ↑ Diabetes insipidus, hyperparathyroidism, renal tubular acidosis
↓ Burns, hyperaldosteronism, adrenal hypofunction, CHF

Mg^+ ↑ Adrenal hypofunction, early stage diabetic acidosis, hypothyroidism, renal failure
↓ Hyperparathyroidism, hyperthyroidism, hyperaldosteronism, malnutrition

PO_4 ↑ Addison's disease, acromegaly, hypoparathyroidism, renal insufficiency, bone metastases, diabetic acidosis
↓ Hyperparathyroidism, diabetes mellitus, renal tubular disorders

K^+ ↑ Hypoaldosteronism, adrenal hypofunction, circulatory failure, diabetes mellitus, renal insufficiency, respiratory acidosis, shock, massive transfusions, hyperparathyroidism
↓ Cushing's syndrome, aldosteronism, alkalosis, hepatic coma, diarrhea, vomiting, CHF, paralytic ileus, diuresis, excessive licorice ingestion

Na^+ ↑ Acute renal failure, CNS disorders, salicylate toxicity, osmotic diuresis, Cushing's syndrome, diabetes insipidus, HHNK, hyperaldosteronism
↓ Adrenal hypofunction, adrenocortical insufficiency, cirrhosis with ascites, Guillain-Barré, burns, SIADH, DKA

(Adapted from Comer, S.R. [1994]. *The ICU Quick Reference*. El Paso, TX: Skidmore-Roth Publishers. Reprinted with permission.)

TABLE 10-2. Lab Findings, Blood Chemistry

Blood Chemistry

Albumin	↑	Diabetic acidosis, hypothyroidism
	↓	Malabsorption, burns, hyperthyroidism, hypocalcemia, chronic liver disease, carcinoma
Alkaline phosphatase	↑	Chronic renal failure, acromegaly, hyperparathyroidism, hyperthyroidism, liver disease, biliary obstruction, bone metastases, mononucleosis, pancreatitis, ulcerative colitis
	↓	Hypothyroidism, pernicious anemia, malnutrition, hypophosphatemia, celiac disease
HCO_3^-	↑	Cushing's syndrome
	↓	Adrenal hypofunction
BUN	↑	Adrenal hypofunction, diabetes mellitus, GI bleeding, renal insufficiency, shock, sepsis, burns
	↓	Acromegaly, liver failure, nephrotic syndrome, overhydration
Creatinine	↑	Diabetes mellitus, adrenal hypofunction, renal insufficiency, prerenal azotemia
Glucose	↑	Acromegaly, Cushing's syndrome, diabetes mellitus, hyperpituitarism, pheochromocytoma, hyperthyroidism, pancreatitis, sepsis, tumors, anoxia, burns, seizures, stress, MI, shock, hyperglycemia, HHNK
	↓	Adrenal hypofunction, hypopituitarism, hypothyroidism, bacterial sepsis, malnutrition, cirrhosis, Reye's syndrome
Total protein	↑	Diabetic acidosis, hypothyroidism, leukemia, multiple myeloma, shock, tuberculosis
	↓	Chronic uncontrolled diabetes mellitus, hyperthyroidism, pancreatitis, hemorrhage, ulcerative colitis, malnutrition, Cushing's syndrome, thyrotoxicosis

(Adapted from Comer, S.R. [1994]. *The ICU Quick Reference*. El Paso, TX: Skidmore-Roth Publishers. Reprinted with permission.)

(continued)

NOTES

TABLE 10-3. Lab Findings, Hematology

Hematology

Hct	↑	Polycythemia, adrenal hypofunction, Cushing's syndrome, dehydration, diabetic acidosis, pheochromocytoma, COPD
	↓	Hemorrhage, anemia, overhydration, DIC, renal failure
Hgb	↑	COPD, polycythemia, Cushing's syndrome, pheochromocytoma, dehydration
	↓	Hemorrhage, anemias, DIC, renal failure, hypopituitarism, hypothyroidism
RBCs	↑	Pituitary tumors, polycythemia, chronic hypoxia
	↓	Adrenal hypofunction, hemolysis, aplastic anemia, hemorrhage, renal failure, DIC

(Adapted from Comer, S.R. [1994]. *The ICU Quick Reference.* El Paso, TX: Skidmore-Roth Publishers. Reprinted with permission.)

 LAB VALUES: CHEMISTRY

TABLE 10-4. Lab Values, Chemistry

A/G ratio	1.2–2.3	
Acetone, serum	negative	
Acid phosphatase	0–0.8	U/L
Albumin	3.8–5.0	g/dL
Alcohol, ethyl	negative	
Alkaline phosphatase	36–120	U/L
Ammonia, plasma	11–35	μmol/L
Amylase, serum	23–85	U/L
Amylase, urine	4–37	U/2 hr
Anion gap	7–17	mEq/L
Bilirubin, direct	0–0.4	mg/dL
Bilirubin, indirect	0–1.1	mg/dL
Bilirubin total	0–1.5	mg/dL
Blood gases, arterial		
pH	7.35–7.45	
$PaCO_2$	35–45	mmHg
Po_2	>80	mmHg
HCO_3^-	22–26	mEq/L
BUN	10–23	μg/dL
Calcium, serum	8.5–10.2	mg/dL
Calcium, urine	30–200	mg/24 hr
Chloride, serum	99–111	mEq/L
Cholesterol, serum	130–300	mg/dL
Cortisol, urine	20–90	μg/24 hr
Cortisol, serum AM	5–25	μg/dL
Cortisol, serum PM	2.5–12.5	μg/dL

(continued)

TABLE 10-4. Lab Values, Chemistry (Continued)

Cortisol stimulation	10–50	μg/dL
Cortisol suppression	0–5	μg/dL
Creatinine clearance		
male	107–139	mL/min
female	87–107	mL/min
Creatinine, serum	0.6–1.3	mg/dL
Ceratinine, urine	1000–2000	mg/24 hr
Ferritin	20–300	ng/mL
Folate, serum	>2.0	ng/mL
Free thyroxine index	1.1–4.8	
Gastric fasting volume	20–100	mL
Gastric fasting pH	1.5–3.5	
Gastric unstim. free acid	0–40	mM
Gastric stim. free acid	10–130	mM
Gastric, 12-hr volume	150–1000	ml
GGTP		
male	11–63	U/L
female	8–35	U/L
Glucose, fasting	70–115	mg/dL
Glucose, 2-hr PP	70–115	mg/dL
IgA	57–414	mg/dL
IgG	568–1483	mg/dL
IgM	20–274	mg/dL
Iron, serum	42–135	μg/dL
Iron binding capacity, total	280–400	μg/dL
Iron saturation	12–50	%
Magnesium	1.8–2.4	mg/dL
Osmolality, serum	280–295	mOsm/kg
Osmolality, urine	500–800	mOsm/L
Phosphorus	2.5–4.9	mg/dL
Potassium, serum	3.5–5.0	mEq/L
Potassium, urine	25–120	mM
Protein, total serum	6.0–8.0	g/dL
Protein, total urine	40–150	mg/24 hr
Salicylate	0–29	mg/dL
Sodium, serum	137–150	mEq/L
Sodium, urine random	40–220	mM
Sodium, urine timed	40–220	mM/L
T_3 uptake	25–40	%
T_4	4.5–12	μg/dL
TSH	0–7	μU/mL
Triglycerides	<210	mg/dL
Uric acid, serum		
male	3.0–7.4	mg/dL
female	2.1–6.2	mg/dL
Vitamin B_{12}	180–960	pg/mL

LAB VALUES: COAGULATION

TABLE 10-5. Lab Values, Coagulation

Bleeding time	4–7	min
Fibrinogen	200–400	mg/dL
Fibrin split products	<10	μg/dL
INR*	2.0–3.0*	
Platelets	150–400	$\times 10^3/mm^3$
Prothrombin time	11–14	sec
PTT	<40	sec
Thrombin clot time	8–10	sec

* The INR (International Normalized Ratio) is intended for patients on stable, long-term oral anticoagulant therapy. Most thromboembolic conditions require the value at 2.0 to 3.0, with values at 2.5 to 3.5 for higher intensity of anticoagulation.

LAB VALUES: CSF

TABLE 10-6. Lab Values, CSF

Pressure	70–180	mm H_2O
Albumin	20–48	mg/dL
Ammonia	25–80	μg/dL
Bicarbonate	20–24	mEq/L
Calcium	2.1–3.0	mEq/L
Cell count	0–5	cells
Chloride	116–122	mEq/L
Glucose	50–80	mg/dL
Magnesium	2.0–2.5	mEq/L
Osmolality	292–297	mOsm/L
Phosphorus	1.2–2.0	mEq/L
Potassium	2.7–3.9	mEq/L
Protein	20–45	mg/dL
Sodium	137–145	mEq/L
Urea	4.4–4.8	mmol/L
Uric acid	0.23–0.27	mg/dL

LAB VALUES: HEMATOLOGY

TABLE 10-7. Lab Values, Hematology

Erythrocyte count (RBC)		
Males	4.7–6.1	$\times\ 10^6/mm^3$
Females	4.2–5.4	$\times\ 10^6/mm^3$
Leukocyte Count (WBC)	4.8–10.8	$\times\ 10^3/mm^3$
Hemoglobin		
Males	14–18	g/dL
Females	12–16	g/dL
Hematocrit		
Males	42–52	%
Females	37–47	%
Reticulocyte Count	0.5–1.5	%
Platelet Count	150–450	$\times\ 10^3/mm^3$
Circulating Eosinophil	150–300	mm^3
Sedimentation Rate		
Males	0–9	mm/hr
Females		
Erythrocyte Indices	0–20	mm/hr
MCV		
Males	80–94	μm^3
Females	81–99	μm^3
MCH	27–32	pg
MCHC	32–36	%
Leukocyte Differential Count		
Neutrophils	40–80	%
Bands	0–6	%
Eosinophils	1–7	%
Basophils	0–1	%
Lymphocytes	24–44	%
Monocytes	3–10	%

NOTES

⬤ LAB VALUES: MYOCARDIAL INFARCTION PROFILE

TABLE 10-8. Lab Values, MI Profile

CPK
Normal males 38–174 IU/L   In MI: Onset of elevation 3–6 h
                          →   Peaks in 12–24 h
Normal females 96–140 IU/L   Stays elevated 3–5 d

CPK-MB
Normal: zero   → In MI: Onset of elevation 2–4 h
                             Peaks in 12–20 h
                             Stays elevated 2–3 d

SGOT
Normal males 7–21 IU/L   In MI: Onset of elevation 12–18 h
                          →   Peaks in 24–48 h
Normal females 6–18 IU/L   Stays elevated 3–4 d

TROPONIN
Healthy individuals have undetectable troponin. Typical MI patients commonly have values greater than 10 ng/mL. Lesser ischemic insults extend to the lower level of detectability (0.4 ng/mL) in a continuous spectrum. Follow serially, comparable to CKMB. Troponin elevation can usually be detected within 4 hours after an acute MI, and can remain elevated to 1–2 weeks.

⬤ LAB VALUES: SPINAL FLUID (see Lab Values: CSF)

NOTES

⬤ LAB VALUES: URINALYSIS

TABLE 10-9. Lab Values, Urine

Specific gravity	1.003–1.030
PH	4.5–7.5
Protein	negative
Leukocytes	negative
Glucose	negative
Ketones	negative
Nitrate	negative
Bilirubin	negative
Blood	negative
Urobilinogen	0–4 mg/24 hr
Epithelial cells	
male	small number
female	large number
WBC	
male	1–5 hpf
female	1–10 hpf
RBC	negative
Casts	negative
Occult blood, fecal	negative
Mono screen	negative
RA screen	negative
RA titer	<1:20
ASO screen	negative
ASO titer	<125 Todd units
VDRL/RPR	nonreactive
Bacteria	negative

24-HOUR URINE

Amylase	280–1100	IU/24 hr
Calcium	100–240	mg/24 hr
Chloride	140–250	mEq/24 hr
Creatinine	1.0–2.0	g/24 hr
Creatinine clearance		
male	100–130	mL/min
	18–25	mg/kg/24-hr total
female	85–125	mL/min
	12–20	mg/kg/24-hr total
Magnesium	24–255	mg/24 hr
Osmolality	500–850	mOsm/kg
Phosphorus	0.9–1.3	g/24 hr
Potassium	26–123	mEq/24 hr
Protein	0–150	mg/24 hr
Sodium	43–217	mEq/24 hr
Urea nitrogen	12–21	g/24 hr
Uric acid	250–750	mg/24 hr

PEAKS AND TROUGHS

TABLE 10-10. Peaks and Troughs

Drug	Therapeutic Levels	When to Sample
Gentamicin	Peak: 4–10 μg/mL Trough: <2.0 μg/ml	Infusion: 30 min Peak: 30 min after infusion complete Trough: <0.5 hr before next dose
Tobramycin	Peak: 4–10 μg/ml Trough: <2.0 μg/mL	Infusion: 30 min Peak: 30 min after infusion complete Trough: <0.5 hr before next dose
Amikacin	Peak: 20–35 μg/mL Trough: <10 μg/mL	Infusion: 30 min Peak: 30 min after infusion complete Trough: <0.5 hr before next dose
Vancomycin	Peak: 25–40 μg/mL Trough: 5–10 μg/mL	Infusion: 1–1.5 hr Peak: 1 hr after infusion complete Trough: <0.5 hr before next dose

N O T E S

THERAPEUTIC DRUG LEVELS

TABLE 10-11. Therapeutic Drug Levels

Anticonvulsants

Carbamazepine	4–12	μg/mL
Klonopin (clonazepam)	40–100	μg/mL
Mysoline (primidone)	7–15	μg/mL
Phenobarbital	15–40	μg/mL
Phenytoin	10–20	μg/mL
Tegretol	8–12	μg/mL
Valproic acid	50–100	μg/mL
Zarontin (ethosuximide)	40–90	μg/mL

Bronchodilators

Aminophylline IV	10–20	μg/mL
Theophylline PO	10–20	μg/mL

Cardiovascular Drugs

Amiodarone	1.0–2.5	μg/mL
Digoxin	0.5–2.0	ng/mL
Lidocaine	1.5–5.0	μg/mL
NAPA	6–20	μg/mL
Procainamide	4–10	μg/mL
Quinidine	2–5	μg/mL

Other Meds

Acetaminophen		
4 hours after ingestion	<150	μg/mL
12 hours after ingestion	<0.5	μg/mL
Amitriptyline	120–250	ng/ml
Desipramine	40–60	ng/ml
Ethanol		
toxic	>2.4	ng/ml
legally drunk	100–200	mg/100 mL
confusion	150–300	mg/100 mL
stupor	250–400	mg/100 mL
coma	350–500	mg/100 mL
death	>500	mg/100 mL
Lithium	0.6–1.5	mEq/mL
Nortriptyline	50–150	ng/mL
Salicylate	15–25	mg/dL
fatal	>60	mg/dL

Note: Drug standards vary considerably between institutions.

P A R T

Miscellaneous

● APACHE II SEVERITY OF DISEASE CLASS SYSTEM

TABLE 11-1. APACHE II Classification System *(continues across spread)*

Physiologic Variable	High Abnormal		
	+4	+3	+2
Temperature, rectal (°C)	≥41°	39–40.9	
Mean arterial pressure, mmHg	≥160	130–159	110–129
Heart rate, ventricular response	≥180	140–179	110–139
Respiratory rate, nonventilated or ventilated	≥50	35–49	
Oxygenation A-aDO$_2$ or PaO$_2$ (mmHg) FiO$_2$ ≥ 0.5 record A-aDO$_2$ FiO$_2$ < 0.5 record only PaO$_2$	≥500	350–499	200–349
Arterial pH	≥7.7	7.6–7.69	
Serum sodium (mmol/L)	≥180	160–179	155–159
Serum potassium (mmol/L)	≥7	6–6.9	
Serum creatinine (mg/100 mL); Double point score for acute renal failure	≥3.5	2–3.4	1.5–1.9
Hematocrit (%)	≥60		50–59.9
White blood count (thousand/mm³)	≥40		20–39.9
Glasgow coma scale (GCS) Score = 15 minus actual GCS			
A Total Acute Physiology Score (APS): Sum of the 12 individual variable points			
Serum HCO$_3$ (venous-mmol/L) [Not preferred, use if no ABGs]	≥52	41–51.9	

Range		Low Abnormal Range			
+1	*0*	*+1*	*+2*	*+3*	*+4*
38.5–38.9	36–38.4	34–35.9	32–33.9	30–31.9	≤29.9
	70–109		50–69		≤49
	70–109		55–69	40–54	≤39
25–34	12–24	10–11	6–9		≤5
	<200 PO_2 > 70	PO_2 61–70		PO_2 55–60	PO_2 < 55
7.5–7.59	7.33–7.49		7.25–7.32	7.15–7.24	<7.15
150–154	130–149		120–129	111–119	≤110
5.5–5.9	3.5–5.4	3–3.4	2.5–2.9		<2.5
	0.6–1.4		<0.6		
46–49.9	30–45.9		20–29.9		<20
15–19.9	3–14.9		1–2.9		<1
32–40.9	22–31.9		18–21.9	15–17.9	<15

B Age Points:
Assign points to age as follows:

Age(yr)	Points
≤44	0
45–54	2
55–64	3
65–74	5
≥75	6

C Chronic Health Points
If the patient has a history of severe organ system insufficiency or is immunocompromised, assign points as follows:

a. for nonoperative or emergency postoperative patients—5 points

or

b. for elective postoperative patients—2 points

Definitions

Organ insufficiency or immunocompromised state must have been evident **prior** to this hospital admission and conform to the following criteria:

Liver: Biopsy-proven cirrhosis and documented portal hypertension; episodes of past upper GI bleeding attributed to portal hypertension; or prior episodes of hepatic failure, encephalopathy, or coma.

Cardiovascular: New York Heart Association Class IV. **Respiratory:** Chronic restrictive, obstructive, or vascular disease resulting in severe exercise restriction, such as unable to climb stairs or perform household duties; or documented chronic hypoxia, hypercapnia, secondary polycythemia, severe pulmonary hypertension (>40 mmHg), or respiratory dependency.

Renal: Receiving chronic dialysis.

Immunocompromised: The patient has received therapy that suppresses resistance to infection, for example, immunosuppression, chemotherapy, radiation, long-term or recent high-dose steroids, or has a disease that is sufficiently advanced to suppress resistance to infection, such as leukemia, lymphoma, AIDS.

APACHE II SCORE

Sum of [A] + [B] + [C]

[A] APS points _____

[B] Age points _____

[C] Chronic Health points _____

Total Apachee II _____

Knaus, W.A., et al. (1995). APACHE II: A Severity of Disease Classification System. *Critical Care Medicine,* 13(10), 818–829.

NOTES

◯ ASSESSMENT CRITERIA

HEENT

Head	Headache, dizziness, syncope
Eyes	Diplopia, exophthalmos, pupil size, eye pain or infection, condition of sclera, visual difficulties, glaucoma, cataracts
Ears	Hearing loss, drainage, tinnitus, ear aches, vertigo
Nose	Discharge, frequent colds and sneezing, nasal obstruction, sinus pain or infection, epistaxis, enlarged, reddened
Throat	Dysphagia, aphagia, red, swollen, sore

Neurologic Assessment

Look for these indicators of neurologic impairment: ability to move extremities, paralysis, involuntary movements, syncope, convulsions, gait, coordination, disturbances regarding hearing and equilibrium, taste, smell, vision, speech, defective memory or thought process, numbness or headache, tingling in extremities, dizziness, weakness.

Cardiovascular Assessment

Assess the following for signs and symptoms of cardiovascular disease: heart rate and rhythm, heart sounds, murmurs. Also note any chest pain and its location, radiation, quality (heavy, burning, squeezing); whether or not it's affected by respirations; time it occurs; and its relationship to exertion, eating, emotions, exposure to cold. Other signs and symptoms include palpitations, exertional dyspnea, orthopnea, presence of cyanosis, edema, phlebitis, temperature of extremities, hypertension, use of cardiac drugs.

Respiratory Assessment

Use these indicators for respiratory impairment: respiratory rate and quality, skin color, chest expansion, use of accessory muscles, pain with respiration, cough (if productive, sputum color), lung sounds, dyspnea, smoker, asthma, emphysema, wheeze, fluid problems.

Gastrointestinal Assessment

Look for these signs and symptoms of GI problems: nausea, vomiting, diarrhea, constipation, dysphagia, loss of appetite, ostomy, bleeding, bowel habits, food intolerance, abdominal distension or tenderness, bowel sounds, last date of any related X-ray films, ulcer, upset stomach, belching.

Genitourinary Assessment

Assess the following for genitourinary impairment: incontinence, urinary tract infections, dysuria, stones, nocturia, hematuria, polyuria, pain, ur-
(continued)

gency, menstrual history, last PAP smear, dysmenorrhea, obstetrical history, testicular pain, change in size of scrotum.

Musculoskeletal Assessment
Look for muscle weakness, back pain, joint pain, stiffness or swelling, rheumatoid or osteoarthritis, gout, bursitis, flat feet, presence or history of fractures, muscle pain or cramping, range of motion, deformities.

Skin Assessment
Evaluate temperature, color, texture, turgor, tendency toward bruising, decubitus, ulcers, rashes, bruises, cuts.

Psychological Assessment
Assess the following psychological indicators: level of consciousness, level of orientation, emotional state (depressed, anxious, euphoric, apprehensive, angry, combative, calm).

◖ BURNS

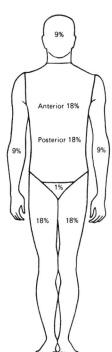

9%

Anterior 18%

Posterior 18%

9%   9%

1%

18%   18%

FIGURE 11-1 Rule of Nines: chart for calculating percentage of body burns in adults.

(continued)

Formulas for Fluid Replacement in Burn Patients

Consensus Formula

Lactated Ringer's solution (or other balanced saline solution): 2–4 ml × body weight × % body surface area (BSA) burned. Half to be given in first 8 hours; remaining half to be given over next 16 hours.

Evans Formula

1. Colloids: 1 ml × kg body weight × % BSA burned
2. Electrolytes (saline): 1 ml × kg body weight × % BSA burned
3. Glucose (5% in water): 2000 ml for insensible loss
   Day 1: Half to be given in first 8 hours; remaining half over next 16 hours.
   Day 2: Half of previous day's colloids and electrolytes; all of insensible fluid replacement.

Maximum of 10,000 mL over 24 hours. Second- and third-degree burns exceeding 50% BSA are calculated on the basis of 50% BSA.

Brooke Army Formula

1. Colloids: 0.5 ml × kg body weight × % BSA burned
2. Electrolytes (lactated Ringer's solution): 1.5 mL × kg body weight × % BSA burned
3. Glucose (5% in water): 2000 ml for insensible loss
   Day 1: Half to be given in first 8 hours; remaining half over next 16 hours.
   Day 2: Half of colloids; half of electrolytes; all of insensible fluid replacement.

Second- and third-degree burns exceeding 50% BSA are calculated on the basis of 50% BSA.

Parkland/Baxter Formula

Lactated Ringer's solution: 4 ml × kg body weight × % BSA burned.
   Day 1: Half to be given in first 8 hours; half to be given over next 16 hours.
   Day 2: Varies. Colloid is added.

Hypertonic Saline Solution

Concentrated solutions of sodium chloride (NaCl) and lactate with concentration of 250–300 mEq of sodium per liter, administered at a rate sufficient to maintain a desired volume of urinary output. Do not increase the infusion rate during the first 8 postburn hours. Serum sodium levels must be monitored closely. Goal: Increase serum sodium level and osmolality to reduce edema and prevent pulmonary complications.

FIGURE 11-2 Formulas for fluid replacement in burn patients. (Adapted from Smeltzer, S.C., & Bare, B.G. [1996]. *Brunner and Suddarth's textbook of medical-surgical nursing* [8th ed.]. Philadelphia: Lippincott-Raven.)

(continued)

TABLE 11-2. Characteristics of Burns According to Depth

Depth of Burn and Causes	Skin Involvement	Symptoms	Wound Appearance	Recuperative Course
SUPERFICIAL (FIRST DEGREE)				
Sunburn Low-intensity flash	Epidermis	Tingling Hyperesthesia (super sensitivity) Pain that is soothed by cooling	Reddened; blanches with pressure Minimal or no edema	Complete recovery within a week Peeling
PARTIAL THICKNESS (SECOND DEGREE)				
Scalds Flash flame	Epidermis and part of dermis	Pain Hyperesthesia Sensitive to cold air	Blistered, mottled red base; broken epidermis; weeping surface Edema	Recovery in 2 to 3 weeks Some scarring and depigmentation Infection may convert it to third degree
FULL THICKNESS (THIRD DEGREE)				
Flame Prolonged exposure to hot liquids Electric current	Epidermis, entire dermis, and sometimes subcutaneous tissue	Pain free Shock Hematuria (blood in the urine) and, possibly, hemolysis (blood cell destruction) Possible entrance and exit wounds (electrical burn)	Dry; pale white, leathery, or charred Broken skin with fat exposed Edema	Eschar sloughs Grafting necessary Scarring and loss of contour and function Loss of digits or extremity possible

NOTES

◖ CENTRAL VENOUS CATHETER REFERENCE

TABLE 11-3. Central Venous Catheters

● **TUNNELED CATHETERS**

Hickman	Has Dacron cuff and clamps.
Broviac	Smaller lumen than Hickman.
	Useful in pediatrics and elderly.
Hickman-Broviac	Combination of the two catheters.
	Used for multiple infusions.

These catheters require flushing with NS before administration of medication, and after administration, NS is again employed in addition to a heparin flush. When the line is not in use, heparin must be instilled at least weekly to maintain patency.

● **PIC LINE (PERIPHERALLY INSERTED CENTRAL CATHETER)**

Long line catheter	Used for patients with poor central access.
	Easily inserted at bedside.
	Lumen smaller than tunneled catheters.

The PIC line requires flushing with NS before administration of medication, and after administration, NS is again employed in addition to a heparin flush.

● **IMPLANTED VENOUS ACCESS PORTS**

Groshong	Implanted like a pacemaker, these catheters contain a
Medi-Port	self-sealing, disk-shaped, silicone septum that is con-
Infuse-A-Port	nected to a metal or plastic port. Useful in patients that
Port-A-Cath	require long-term scheduled infusions.

These ports require flushing with NS before administration of a medication, and after administration, NS is again employed in addition to a heparin flush. When the port is not in use, it must be flushed every 4 weeks with NS and heparin to prevent clot formation.

◖ DRUG CLASSIFICATIONS

Class I antiarrhythmics	Sodium blockade
Class II antiarrhythmics	Beta blockade
Class III antiarrhythmics	Potassium blockade
Class IV antiarrhythmics	Calcium channel blockers

◯ DRUG HINTS

- ACE (angiotensin converting enzyme) inhibitors prevent conversion of angiotensin I to angiotensin II. They are used for treatment of hypertension and as an unloading agent in heart failure.

- Drugs ending in *"pril"* (eg, captopril) are ACE inhibitors.

- Inotropic agents increase muscular contractility. **REMEMBER: "iron" = strength.**

- Chronotropic agents increase heart rate.

- Dromotropic agents speed conduction.

- Pressors increase blood supply by vasoconstriction.

- α-Adrenergic receptor stimulators
  - α_1 agents are used for vasoconstriction, inotropic action.
  - α_2 agents are used for vasoconstriction.

- β-Adrenergic receptor stimulators
  - β_1 agents are chronotropic and inotropic.
  - β_2 agents are used for vasodilation and bronchial relaxation.

- Catecholamines
  - Norepinephrine acts on α-adrenergic receptors.
  - Dopamine is a precursor of norepinephrine.
  - Epinephrine acts on α- and β-adrenergic receptors.
  - Isoproterenol is a synthetic catecholamine that acts on β-adrenergic receptors.

- Adrenergic ("stimulator") agents are also known as sympathomimetic. Adrenergic fibers liberate norepinephrine, causing vasoconstriction of arterioles in the skin and splanchnic area, resulting in an increase in blood pressure.

- β-Adrenergic receptors cause increased heart rate, increased conduction velocity, vasodilation of arterioles supplying skeletal muscle, bronchial relaxation, and relaxation of GI and uterine smooth muscle. β-Adrenergic receptors are of two types: β_1 receptors are located primarily in the heart and mediate actions there, whereas β_2 receptors mediate the actions of catecholamines on the bronchioles of the lungs and arterial smooth muscle.

REMEMBER: β_1 receptors work on the heart: your body has **one** heart. β_2 receptors work primarily on the lungs: your body has **two** lungs.
  - Cholinergic agents are also known as parasympathomimetic. Cholinergic fibers liberate acetylcholine.

  - Drugs that can be diluted and put down an ET tube make up the pneumonic **NAVEL: N**arcan **a**tropine **V**alium **e**pinephrine **l**idocaine.

MRSA ERADICATION PROTOCOL*

1. The patient with methicillin-resistant *Staphylococcus aureus* should be placed in contact isolation. Isolation should continue until the patient has one set of negative cultures.

2. For 5 days give:

a. Sulfamethoxazole-trimethoprim (Bactrim), 2 single-strength tablets BID; or minocycline, 100 mg BID

b. Rifampin, 300 mg BID

c. Bacitracin or mupirocin ointment to the anterior nasal vestibule, BID

d. Daily bath with chlorhexidine solution.

3. After the 5th day of medications, the patient's bed and bed area should be manually cleaned with disinfectant.

4. Follow-up surveillance cultures should be taken to determine success of the protocol. Three culture swabs should be used: one to culture anterior nares, one for both axilla, and one for both groin. In addition, any open wound should be cultured.

The drug regimen is not being recommended for clinical illnesses. The regimen should be very safe, but it needs to be determined if there is a reason it should not be given (eg, allergy to sulfa drugs or renal failure).

This protocol varies from institution to institution.

ORGAN DONATION

Criteria

• Age of donor ranges from newborn to 65 years. However, an individual of any age with a cardiorespiratory death may be a candidate for tissue and eye donation.

• Donor must be brain dead by legal and medical criteria (see below).

• Donor must have intact heartbeat and circulation.

• Apneic donors must be on ventilator.

• There must be absence of:
  • Sepsis or transmissible disease
  • Cancer, except primary brain tumor
  • Insulin-dependent diabetes
  • Chronic, uncontrolled hypertension

Brain Death Criteria

• Cause of condition is known.

• Diagnosis is made in absence of hypothermia (temperature <32.2°C) and central nervous system depressants.

- Patient is areflexic except for simple spinal cord reflexes; pupillary, extraocular, corneal, gag, and cough reflexes are absent.

- No spontaneous respiration is present (see apnea test below).

- Condition is irreversible.

    Duration of observation depends on clinical judgment; 12 hours is recommended when an irreversible condition is well established and no confirmatory test; 24 hours is recommended for anoxic brain damage and no confirmatory test.

- EEG (if performed) is flat.

- Blood flow, as indicated by cerebral radionuclide scan or arteriogram (if performed), is absent.

Apnea Test

- Preoxygenate patient.

- Disconnect ventilator, give O_2 at 8 to 12 L/min by tracheal cannula. Observe for spontaneous respirations.

- After 10 minutes, draw ABG. PCO_2 must be >60 mmHg for accurate test.

- Reconnect the ventilator.

- Patient is apneic if PCO_2 is >60 mmHg and there is no respiratory movement.

- If hypotension and/or arrhythmia develop during test, immediately reconnect the ventilator and consider other confirmatory test.

For more information on organ donation, call 1-800-24-DONOR (243-6667). This line is staffed 24 hours a day by organ procurement professionals for the referral of potential organ donors by physicians and other health care professionals. This hotline is also available to health care personnel for the acquisition of general information concerning organ donation and the procurement of organs for transplantation.

NOTES

⬤ PAIN MANAGEMENT

TABLE 11-4. Pain Management

	Analgesia	Anxiety Control	Amnesia	Other
Opiates fentanyl morphine sulfate demerol codeine	Good	Fair	None	Suppresses dyspnea sensation
Benzodiazepines diazepam lorazepam midazolam	None	Good	Variable	Raises seizure threshold
Antipsychotics haloperidol chlorpromazine fluphenazine	None	Moderate	None	
Propofol	None	Good	Dose dependent	Used for mechanically ventilated patients

⬤ PAP SMEAR CLASSIFICATIONS

Class 1	Normal cells
Class 2	Atypical cells, probably normal
Class 3	Doubtful, may be malignant
Class 4	Probably malignant
Class 5	Definite malignancy

NOTES

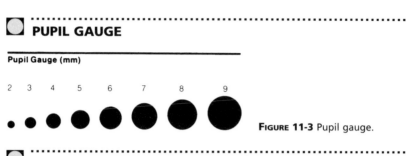

⬤ PUPIL GAUGE

Pupil Gauge (mm)

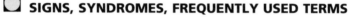

2   3   4   5   6   7   8   9

Figure 11-3 Pupil gauge.

⬤ SIGNS, SYNDROMES, FREQUENTLY USED TERMS

Babinski's Reflex

Babinski's reflex is dorsiflexion of big toe upon scratching bottom of foot. It indicates upper motor neuron dysfunction.

Battle's Sign

Battle's sign is ecchymosis behind the ear and is associated with basilar skull fracture.

Brudzinski's Sign

Brudzinski's sign is flexion of the neck causing flexion of the legs. It is seen in meningitis (see also Kernig's Sign).

Chvostek's Sign

Chvostek's sign is evidenced by tapping over the facial nerve causing facial twitching in hypocalcemic state (see also Trousseau's Sign).

Cullen's Sign

Cullen's sign is bluish color around the umbilicus seen in hemorrhagic pancreatitis.

Fremitus

Fremitus is a vibration palpated when patient speaks. Sound is best conducted through solid material; therefore, fremitus is increased in atelectasis, lung tumors. Sound is more poorly conducted through fluid and air; therefore, fremitus is decreased in pneumothorax, pleural effusions, emphysema.

Grey Turner's Sign

Grey Turner's sign is ecchymosis in the flank associated with retroperitoneal bleeding.

Homans's Sign

Homans's sign is calf pain with dorsiflexion of the foot associated with deep vein thrombosis.

(continued)

Janeway Lesions

Janeway lesions are slightly raised, irregular, nontender, erythematous lesions on palms and soles; they are a possible indication of infective endocarditis.

Kehr's Sign

Kehr's sign is seen in 50% of splenic injuries. Pain is referred to left shoulder.

Kerley's B Lines

Kerley's B lines are seen on chest X-ray films and are indicative of pulmonary edema.

Kernig's Sign

Kernig's sign is seen with thigh flexed at right angle: complete extension of the leg is not possible. It is seen in meningitis.

McBurney's Point

McBurney's point is located one-third the distance from the anterior superior iliac spine to the umbilicus. McBurney's sign is tenderness of the site and is associated with appendicitis.

Murphy's Sign

Murphy's sign is severe pain and inspiratory arrest with palpation of the right upper quadrant. It is associated with cholecystitis.

Psoas Sign

With psoas sign, extension and elevation of the right leg produces pain in cases of inflammation of the psoas muscle. The sign is positive with appendicitis.

Quincke's Sign

Quincke's sign is alternating blushing and blanching of the fingernail bed following light compression. It is seen in aortic regurgitation.

Roth's Spots

Roth's spots are round or oval white spots seen in the retina; they are a possible indication of subacute bacterial endocarditis.

Romberg's Sign

Romberg's sign is seen when patient stands with feet close together and eyes closed: unsteadiness is associated with cerebellar damage.

(continued)

Somogyi Effect

Somogyi effect is rebound hyperglycemia (insulin causing high glucose).

Trousseau's Sign

Trousseau's sign is carpopedal spasm following restriction of circulation to arm by BP cuff. It is indicative of hypocalcemia (see also Chvostek's Sign).

NOTES

○ TED HOSE SIZING CHART

TABLE 11-5. Knee High

Calf Circumference	10"	11"	12"	13"	14"	15"	16"	17"	18"	19"
Length to Knee										
13"	S	S	S	S	S	M	M	M	XL	XL
14"	S	S	S	S	M	M	M	L	XL	XL
15"	S	S	S	M	M	M	L	L	XL	XL
16"	S	S	S	M	M	M	L	L	XL	XL
17"	S	S	M	M	M	M	L	L	XL	XL
18"	S	M	M	M	M	L	L	L	XL	XL
19"	M	M	M	M	M	L	L	XL	XL	XL

TABLE 11-6. Thigh High*

Calf Circumference	10"	11"	12"	13"	14"	15"	16"	17"	18"	19"
Length to Gluteal Fold										
26"	S	S	S	S	S	S	M	M	XL	XL
27"	S	S	S	S	S	M	M	L	XL	XL
28"	S	S	S	S	M	M	M	L	XL	XL
29"	S	S	S	M	M	M	L	L	XL	XL
30"	S	S	S	M	M	M	L	L	XL	XL
31"	S	S	M	M	M	M	L	L	XL	XL
32"	S	S	M	M	M	L	L	L	XL	XL
33"	S	M	M	M	L	L	L	L	XL	XL

*Do not apply if upper thigh circumference exceeds 32 in.

⬤ **UNIVERSAL PRECAUTIONS**

Universal Precautions
OSHA Guidelines for Occupational Exposure
Universal precautions for use with ALL patients
(Adapted from the CDC)

1. Wash hands after contact with body substances, i.e., urine, sputum, blood, etc., before invasive procedures and before eating or preparing food.
2. Wear gloves for direct hand contact with patient body substances (blood, urine, sputum, etc.), mucous membranes, non-intact skin, and when doing dressing changes.
3. Wear paper isolation gown or plastic apron if soiling with any body substance is likely.
4. When performing procedures that may result in splashing of patient body fluids (i.e., tracheal suctioning, wound irrigation, endoscopy) wear paper isolation gown or plastic apron, mask, and clear plastic goggles for eye and mouth protection.
5. Used needles shall not be bent, broken, recapped or otherwise manipulated by hand. ONE-HANDED RECAPPING by the blood gas technician is, however, acceptable.
6. Dispose of needles and sharps in plastic needle/sharps containers provided for that purpose.
7. If exposure to blood or body fluids occurs, remove the body substance by washing hands, face, arms, or other body area affected. IMMEDIATELY report the exposure to your supervisor.
8. Treat all patient specimens as potentially infective.
9. Clean up spills of blood/body fluids with a hospital grade disinfectant, used at manufacturer's recommended dilution. For large spills, notify environmental services immediately. They have the special equipment and information needed to handle such spills.
10. Although saliva HAS NOT been implicated in the transmission of HIV, minimize the need for mouth-to-mouth resuscitation by using one-way valve mouthpieces, resuscitation bags or other ventilation devices in CPR situations.

FIGURE 11-4 Universal precautions. (Adapted from the Centers for Disease Control. Oakes, D. [1994]. *Clinical practitioner's guide to respiratory care.* Old Towne, Maine: Health Educator Publications.)

Clinical Notes

- The collection of arterial blood gases has been singled out by the CDC as a procedure wherein recapping of needles is often a medical necessity. However, never recap by holding the cap in one hand and pushing the needle into the cap. When you must recap, lay the cap down on a flat surface and insert the needle into the cap, picking it up off the surface without touching the cap with your other hand. Once you have done this, you can point the needle to the ceiling and secure the cap onto the hub, touching only the base of the cap.
- As an alternative to the above, you can place the cap into the plastic shroud that the 3 ml syringes come in. The shroud can be held or left standing on a flat surface, providing a holder for the cap and allowing the needle to be re-capped safely.
- Always wear the equipment that is needed to avoid contact of any kind with blood or other body fluids (e.g. gloves when handling contaminated circuits).
- Wash hands between patients even if using gloves. Never re-use gloves from patient to patient. Always wash hands even after removal of gloves.
- Use the Faceshields (masks with plastic eye protection built in) when faced with any possibility of splashing or splattering body fluid into your face in other circumstances. The regular surgical masks offer less protection to penetration by fluids.
- Be sure to use the special white masks (3M PN #1814 Healthcare Particulate Respirator) when giving pentamidine or working with active TB patients. Use eye protection in addition when there is any threat of splashing into your face.
- Normal prescription eyewear serves as protective equipment only if fitted with side shields.
- Procedures should always be done in such a manner as to minimize the splashing or spraying of blood and body fluids.

FIGURE 11-4 (Continued)

Additional Credits*

Part 1

Figs. 1-1, 1-2, 1-8, 1-11, 1-12, 1-13, 1-14, 1-16, 1-17, 1-19, 1-22, 1-26: Hudak, C.M., Gallo, B.M., Morton, P.G. (1998). *Critical Care Nursing*, 7th ed. Philadelphia: Lippincott-Raven.

Figs. 1-4, 1-5, 1-6, 1-7, 1-9, 1-18, and Table 1-2: Hickey, J.V. (1997). *The Clinical Practice of Neurological and Neurosurgical Nursing*, 4th ed. Philadelphia: Lippincott-Raven.

Fig. 1-21: Smeltzer, S.C., Bare, B.G. (1996). *Brunner and Suddarth's Textbook of Medical-Surgical Nursing*, 8th ed. Philadelphia: Lippincott-Raven.

Figs. 1-27, 1-28, 1-29, 1-33: Bates, B. (1995). *A Guide to Physical Examination and History Taking*, 6th ed. Philadelphia: J.B. Lippincott.

Part 2

Fig. 2-50: Bullock, B.L. (1996). *Pathophysiology: Adaptations and Alterations in Function*, 4th ed. Philadelphia: Lippincott-Raven.

Figs. 2-3, 2-30, 2-31, 2-32, 2-33, 2-34, 2-46, 2-49: Hudak, C.M., Gallo, B.M., Morton, P.G. (1998). *Critical Care Nursing*, 7th ed. Philadelphia: Lippincott-Raven.

Figs. 2-11, 2-47, 2-51, 2-52: Woods, S.L., Froelicher, E.S., Halpenny, C.J., Motzer, S.U. (1995). *Cardiac Nursing*, 3rd ed. Philadelphia: J.B. Lippincott.

Fig. 2-28: Smeltzer, S.C., Bare, B.G. (1996). *Brunner and Suddarth's Textbook of Medical-Surgical Nursing*, 8th ed. Philadelphia: Lippincott-Raven.

Fig. 2-13: Porth C.M. (1994). *Pathophysiology: Concepts of Altered Health States*, 4th ed. Philadelphia: J.B. Lippincott.

Figs. 2-17, 2-18, 2-19: Huff, J. (1997). *ECG Workout*, 3rd ed. Philadelphia: Lippincott-Raven.

Part 3

Figs. 3-2, 3-9, 3-10, 3-11, 3-13: Bullock, B.L. (1996). *Pathophysiology: Adaptations and Alterations in Function*, 4th ed. Philadelphia: Lippincott-Raven.

Figs. 3-3, 3-31: Bates, B. (1995). *A Guide to Physical Examination and History Taking*, 6th ed. Philadelphia: J.B. Lippincott.

Figs. 3-4, 3-16, 3-20, 3-21, 3-22, 3-23, 3-24, 3-26, 3-27, 3-28, 3-29, 3-30 and Table 3-2: Hudak, C.M., Gallo, B.M., Morton, P.G. (1998). *Critical Care Nursing*, 7th ed. Philadelphia: Lippincott-Raven.

* *These figures and tables © Lippincott Williams & Wilkins. No adaptations were made to these figures and tables for publication in this book.*

Figs. 3-7, 3-34: Smeltzer, S.C., Bare, B.G. (1996). *Brunner and Suddarth's Textbook of Medical-Surgical Nursing*, 8th ed. Philadelphia: Lippincott-Raven.

Table 3-8. Burton, G.G., Hodgkin, J.E., Ward, J.J., Hess, D., Pilbeam, S.P., Tietsort, J. (1997). *Respiratory Care: A Guide to Clinical Practice*, 4th ed. Philadelphia: Lippincott-Raven.

Part 4

Figs. 4-1, 4-14: Hudak, C.M., Gallo, B.M., Morton, P.G. (1998). *Critical Care Nursing*, 7th ed. Philadelphia: Lippincott-Raven.

Figs. 4-4, 4-7, 4-10: Taylor, C., Lillis, C., & LeMone, P. (1997). *The Art & Science of Nursing Care*, 3rd ed. Philadelphia: Lippincott-Raven.

Figs. 4-9, 4-12, 4-13, 4-15: Smeltzer, S.C., Bare, B.G. (1996). *Brunner and Suddarth's Textbook of Medical-Surgical Nursing*, 8th ed. Philadelphia: Lippincott-Raven.

Part 5

Fig. 5-5: Bullock, B.L. (1996). *Pathophysiology: Adaptations and Alterations in Function*, 4th ed. Philadelphia: Lippincott-Raven.

Figs. 5-6, 5-7, 5-8: Smeltzer, S.C., Bare, B.G. (1996). *Brunner and Suddarth's Textbook of Medical-Surgical Nursing*, 8th ed. Philadelphia: Lippincott-Raven.

Fig. 5-10, Table 5-1: Hudak, C.M., Gallo, B.M., Morton, P.G. (1998). *Critical Care Nursing*, 7th ed. Philadelphia: Lippincott-Raven.

Part 6

Table 6-1: Hudak, C.M., Gallo, B.M., Morton, P.G. (1998). *Critical Care Nursing*, 7th ed. Philadelphia: Lippincott-Raven.

Part 7

Fig. 7-4: Bullock, B.L. (1996). *Pathophysiology: Adaptations and Alterations in Function*, 4th ed. Philadelphia: Lippincott-Raven.

Fig. 7-5: Hudak, C.M., Gallo, B.M., Morton, P.G. (1998). *Critical Care Nursing*, 7th ed. Philadelphia: Lippincott-Raven.

Fig. 7-2: Porth C.M. (1994). *Pathophysiology: Concepts of Altered Health States*, 4th ed. Philadelphia: J.B. Lippincott.

Part 9

Table 9-1: Malseed, R.T., Goldstein, F.J., Balkon N. (1995). *Pharmacology: Drug Therapy and Nursing Management*, 4th ed. Philadelphia: J.B. Lippincott.

Part 11

Fig. 11-1 and Table 11-2: Smeltzer, S.C., Bare, B.G. (1996). *Brunner and Suddarth's Textbook of Medical-Surgical Nursing*, 8th ed. Philadelphia: Lippincott-Raven.

Fig. 11-3: Hickey, J.V. (1997). *The Clinical Practice of Neurological and Neurosurgical Nursing*, 4th ed. Philadelphia: Lippincott-Raven.

Index